KU-483-019

Health communication
Theory and practice

Dianne Berry

1958227

LIBRARY

ACC. No 3606785	DEPT.
CLASS No.	

UNIVERSITY
OF CHESTER

Open University Press

Open University Press
McGraw-Hill Education
McGraw-Hill House
Shoppenhangers Road
Maidenhead
Berkshire
England
SL6 2QL

email: enquiries@openup.co.uk
world wide web: www.openup.co.uk

and Two Penn Plaza, New York, NY 10121-2289, USA

© Dianne Berry 2007

All rights reserved. Except for the quotation of short passages for the purposes of
criticism and review, no part of this publication may be reproduced, stored in a
retrieval system, or transmitted, in any form, or by any means, electronic, mechanical,
photocopying, recording or otherwise, without the prior written permission of the
publisher or a licence from the Copyright Licensing Agency Limited. Details of
such licences (for reprographic reproduction) may be obtained from the Copyright
Licensing Agency Ltd of 90 Tottenham Court Road, London, W1T 4LP.

A catalogue record of this book is available from the British Library

ISBN-10 0 335 21870 9 (pb)   0 335 21871 7 (hb)

ISBN-13 978 0335 21870 7 (pb)   978 0335 21871 4 (hb)

Library of Congress Cataloging-in-Publication Data
CIP data has been applied for

Typeset by RefineCatch Ltd, Bungay, Suffolk
Printed in Poland by OZGraf S.A.
www.polskabook.pl

Accession no.
36061785

Health communication *WITHDRAWN*

University of
Chester

ARROWE PARK
LIBRARY

This book is to be returned on or before the last date stamped
below. Overdue charges will be incurred by the late return of
books.

- 8 JUL 2009

CANCELLED

- 4 JAN 2010

CANCELLED

WITHDRAWN

LIBRARY
0151 604 7291

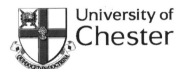

Health psychology

Series editors:
Sheila Payne and Sandra Horn

Contents

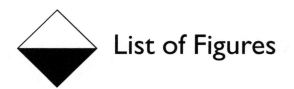 # List of Figures

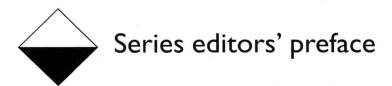

Series editors' preface

This series of books in health psychology is celebrating its tenth anniversary with the publication of this book. This has been a time of rapid growth in the popularity of health psychology as a taught subject at undergraduate and postgraduate level in universities around the world. In addition, health psychology is also emerging strongly as an important 'voice' in psychology with influential things to say about health promotion, healthcare services and health experiences for those with acute and chronic conditions. Concerned as it is with the application of psychological theories and models to the promotion and maintenance of health and the individual and interpersonal aspects of adaptive behaviour in illness and disability, health psychology has a wide remit. Health psychologists are working in many areas including influencing healthcare policies at national level, investigating new interventions and health behaviours, and working directly with clients or in multidisciplinary teams to deliver good psychological care for those facing illness and impairment. Our book series was designed to support postgraduate and post-qualification studies in psychology, nursing, medicine and paramedical sciences and health psychology units in the undergraduate curriculum.

We are delighted that Professor Dianne Berry has contributed a second book to our series. This time she has drawn on her extensive research experience to consider communication in healthcare contexts. It is hard to believe that just two decades ago communication was not even included as a core topic for health professionals. We have seen a remarkable, and in our view appropriate, recognition of the central importance of communication in all aspects of healthcare. Professor Berry is not only an expert in communication but also an expert communicator herself. The book is written with great clarity but with an admirable economy of expression which is likely to be of benefit to students. The text covers types of communication, theoretical models and the research evidence in healthcare. She acknowledges that healthcare communication is particularly difficult in certain situations such as during the delivery of bad news of diagnostic and prognostic information. There are also certain groups of people such as children, older people and those with learning difficulty where communication behaviours need special attention. Most health professionals now are required to undergo communication skills training, and this forms the focus of her final chapter. It may be assumed that communication is now well recognized and taught to health professionals but it still forms one of the major reasons for dissatisfaction and complaints by patients using health services. The insights and evidence from health psychology can contribute to improving communication in healthcare and therefore the experience of patients and their families. We warmly welcome readers to this fine new book.

Sheila Payne and Sandra Horn
Series Editors

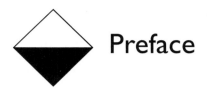# Preface

Two years ago, I published a book on risk communication and health. When I came to the end of it, I realized that there was still much more that needed to be said about other aspects of health communication. This realization, and its ready acceptance by others, led to the decision to write the current book.

I have been working in the area of health communication for about 20 years now, and I am still deeply interested in it. During this period, the importance of effective health communication has become increasingly recognized, yet we are still exposed to numerous examples of poor and inadequate health communications. These may be from our personal dealings with healthcare providers of various sorts, or they may be via the media and other similar channels. Rarely a week goes by when the media do not inform us about some new health scare, and all too often the information is misleading, confusing, or poorly presented in some other way.

The topic of communication has always fascinated me. Maybe this is why all of my school reports mentioned the fact that I talked too much; from my first report, when I was 5, that referred to me as a 'chatterbox', to the last one when I was 16, which stated that I was 'far too gregarious'. The descriptors changed over the years, but the basic message was the same.

Communication is a fundamental process. In fact, it is virtually impossible not to communicate at all; even a non-response sends a message. On the one hand, communication seems effortless; yet things can easily go wrong, sometimes with serious consequences. A breakdown of communication has often been said to be the cause of personal relationships breaking up, particularly after some serious, challenging event has occurred, such as the loss of a child. In such cases two, or a small number of, people's lives may be adversely affected. At another level, however, large numbers of people can be adversely affected by inadequate communication that takes place as part of official public health campaigns or biased and sensationalized media reports of health-related matters.

Health is an area where effective communication is particularly important, as good communication contributes to virtually all aspects of healthcare. There is now a substantial body of evidence to show that patients who are dealt with by healthcare providers with good communication skills have better health outcomes. The converse, ineffective communication, whether at the individual health professional or wider public health level, can lead to patients not even engaging with the healthcare system, refusing to follow recommended advice or to adhere to treatment regimens and failing to cope with the psychological consequences of their illness.

This book draws on material from several different disciplines, including psychology, sociology, health, medicine, pharmacy, statistics and business and management. After providing a brief introduction to health communication and the importance of effective communication, it looks in more detail at the processes that underlie human communication. It also covers the main theories and models that have been proposed to explain how we communicate. The book looks at communication between the different parties involved in the healthcare process and then considers the challenging topics of communicating in difficult circumstances and with people with particular problems. The final sections cover communication at the health promotion/public health level, and how best to improve communication skills. I hope that it will be of interest to fellow researchers, practitioners and students who want to know more about the communication of information in health.

Although this is a single-authored text, a number of others have contributed to my thinking in this area. First, a long-standing colleague and now dear friend, Fiorella de Rosis from the University of Bari in Italy invited me to join a European Commission project on developing an intelligent drug prescription system. She and her colleagues worked with my group in Oxford, and then Reading, in developing and evaluating the explanations that were generated by the system for users. Following this, Irene Michas and I received funding from the UK's Medical Research Council to take the work further. The particular focus of the project was investigating the effects of providing people with different information, in different forms, about medication side effects. Elisabetta Bersellini, who has continued to work with me for the past 10 years, was employed as the research fellow. I am very grateful to Beba (as she is known) for all that she has contributed over this time. More recently, I have also worked with several other research assistants and PhD students in Reading – including Hedwig Natter and Natalie Lynch – and some of their work is referred to in the chapters that follow. I have also collaborated with researchers in other disciplines in Reading, primarily Molly Courtenay and Chris Newdick, and with clinicians at the local Royal Berkshire and Battle Hospitals Trust, particularly Tony Bradlow. One research collaboration that has been particularly productive over the past five years has involved my working with Theo Raynor and Peter Knapp from the University of Leeds. I very much appreciate their contributions to my thinking in this area. Finally, I am very grateful to my personal assistant, Susan Addison, for her professionalism, friendship, and her constant help and support.

When writing a preface, one always tends to leave the most personal thanks to last. I am following this tradition but, as is often the case, last in no way implies least. I am particularly grateful to my husband, John Harris, and to my children, Marc and Kate Berry, for their encouragement and support. Finally, I am especially grateful to my parents, Jean and Maurice Broadfield, for their continuing help and support. Without this, I would never have been able to establish my career while raising a young family, and would not have been in the position, some years later, to write this book.

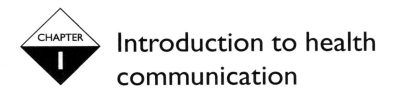

Introduction to health communication

> Information is fundamental to choice and making informed decisions. Without information, there is no choice. Information helps knowledge and understanding. It gives patients the power and confidence to engage as partners with their health service.
>
> (Department of Health, 2004, p. 2)

Communication is the means by which such information is imparted and shared with others. Put more formally, it is the transfer of information between a source and one or more receivers; a process of sharing meanings, using a set of common rules (Northouse and Northouse, 1998). We communicate information in many different ways. In humans, it is frequently done through spoken and/or written language, but non-verbal communication also plays a significant role in our interactions. Thus, our body posture, our expressions, and even the clothes we wear also contribute to the messages that we give out. We constantly communicate information, intentionally or unintentionally, about our perceptions, intentions and feelings, as well as about our very identity. People cannot not communicate. Even saying or doing nothing conveys a message. Not smiling or laughing at an appropriate time can send just as strong a signal as smiling or laughing. Novelist, Anita Brookner, epitomizes this in her award-winning *Hotel du Lac*, when the main male character says, 'for someone who is not speaking you are giving away volumes of information' (Brookner, 1984, p. 76).

Communication is central to our everyday functioning and can be the very essence of the human condition (Hargie and Dickson, 2004). As so aptly put by Hybels and Weaver (1998, p. 5), 'To live is to communicate. To communicate is to enjoy life more fully'. Without the capacity for sophisticated channels for sharing our knowledge, both within and between generations, our advanced civilization would not exist (Hargie and Dixon, 2004).

At its simplest level, communication requires a sender, a message, a receiver and a channel of communication. However, any communicative event is enormously complex; senders are often receivers, and multiple and contradictory messages may be being sent via different channels. We have all experienced situations where a person says one thing but their tone of voice or body language indicates that they actually believe something else. Communication is social in a variety of ways. It frequently involves relations between people and requires people to have a shared understanding of what particular sounds, words and gestures mean. It is the primary means by which people influence others and, in turn, are influenced by them. In such interpersonal settings, it is typically an ongoing and dynamic, or transactional, process. However, human communication may also occur in other settings. It is often necessary to impart information to the wider public in order to reach mass audiences, such as in public health campaigns. As we will see later in this book, effective health promotion campaigns require different communication skills and strategies from those involved in one-to-one or small-group interactions. Human communication does not always involve sharing information with others, however. It can involve communication that takes place solely within a person, through the use of processes such as reflection. Thus, in many everyday situations, we need to solve problems by thinking through alternative courses of action, or we need to monitor the results of our interactions with others.

This book is specifically concerned with health communication: it is about all aspects of human communication that relate to health. More formally, health communication has been defined as referring to 'any type of human communication whose content is concerned with health' (Rogers, 1996, p. 15), where the focus is on health-related transactions and the factors that influence these. Thus, this book will cover a wide range of topics, including the different forms of communication that humans have at their disposal, and the theories and models that have been formulated to account for these; the different types of communication between the various 'players' in the healthcare process, be they patients, carers, health professionals, or others; the issues raised by communicating with particular 'populations' or in difficult circumstances; the challenge of communicating with wider mass audiences in order to promote better health; and different ways of improving health communication skills.

The centrality of communication in health

As should already be becoming clear, effective communication is central to our ability to function as a member of society. It is a key aspect of all relationships, whether these occur in family, educational, work or social settings. Indeed, when such relationships break down or become stressful, the central complaint frequently relates to poor communication. How often do we hear phrases such as 'I tried to explain but he just wouldn't listen' or 'she keeps it all bottled up'? The area of healthcare is no exception. As we will see, communication problems can occur at many different levels.

Effective communication is now generally acknowledged to be central to effective healthcare. It is no longer seen as an add-on extra; rather it is recognized by many as being at the heart of patient care – as playing a pivotal role. As Kreps et al. (1998) noted, communication is pervasive in creating, gathering and sharing health information. It is a central human process that enables individual and collective adaptation to health risks at many different levels (Kreps, 2003).

A significant event in relation to health communication in the UK was the publication of the Patients' Charter (Department of Health, 1992), which informed patients that they had a right to be given a clear explanation of any treatment proposed, including any risks involved and alternatives to the recommended treatment. At a similar time, an international conference on health communication produced the 'Toronto Consensus Statement' on the relationship between communication practices and health outcomes (Simpson et al., 1991). The statement made eight key points:

1 Communication problems in medical practice are important and common.
2 Patient anxiety and dissatisfaction are related to uncertainty and lack of information, explanation and feedback.
3 Doctors often misperceive the amount and type of information that patients want to receive.
4 Improved quality of clinical communication is related to positive health outcomes.
5 Explaining and understanding patient concerns, even when they cannot be resolved, results in a fall in anxiety.
6 Greater participation by the patient in the encounter improves satisfaction, compliance and treatment outcomes.
7 The level of psychological distress in patients with serious illness is less when they perceive themselves to have received adequate information.
8 Beneficial clinical communication is routinely possible in clinical practice and can be achieved during normal clinical encounters, without unduly prolonging them, provided that the clinician has learned the relevant techniques.

There is now a substantial body of evidence to show that healthcare providers who communicate well with patients are more likely to secure positive outcomes for patients, themselves and others. Thus, they are more likely to make more accurate and comprehensive diagnoses, to detect emotional distress in patients, to have patients who are more satisfied with their care and less anxious, and who agree with and follow the advice given (e.g. Lloyd and Bor, 1996). In addition, patients who are dealt with by professionals with good communication skills have been shown to have improved health indices and recovery rates (e.g. Davis and Fallowfield, 1994; Greenfield et al. 1985; Ong et al., 1995). Thus, in what is now cited as a classic series of studies by Greenfield et al. (1985), informing and involving patients in their cases led to significant reductions in blood pressure and improvements in diabetic control that were comparable with the introduction of a new drug. Similar findings have been reported in more recent studies (e.g. Dulmen and Bensing, 2001; Roter, 2000; Stewart, 1995; Williams et al., 1998). As Schofield (2004) noted, 'effective communication was a drug that could be prescribed!' (p. xix).

However, we also know that such positive outcomes are not always obtained. Whereas effective communication has been shown to have the above beneficial effects, ineffective communication can lead to a whole range of negative outcomes. These include, patients not engaging with the health service when they should, refusing to follow recommended health behaviours and undergo necessary treatment, failing to adhere to treatment regimens, or failing to cope with their own or another's illness. In extreme cases, poor communication can lead to psychological damage, physical harm, litigation or, at worst, death (e.g. MacDonald, 2004). In a nutshell, as noted by Pettigrew and Logan (1987), communication promotes both health and illness in society, and makes the system run at optimal or marginal effectiveness.

The emphasis must therefore be on *effective* communication, rather than on communication per se. We need to impart the right information, to the right people, in the right way, at the right time. Simply providing more information per se cannot be a goal in itself. Communication needs to be patient centred and informative, and needs to promote trust and confidence. As MacDonald (2004) noted, good communication between patients and medical staff is important from the very first encounter, because it forms the basis of all future transactions. Thus, in line with this, the theme of 'effective communication', and the factors that are involved in this and how it might best be achieved, are central to this book and will run throughout the chapters that follow.

Different forms of communication and theories, and models to account for these

As mentioned earlier, many of our communications involve the use of language (either spoken or written). It is our capacity for these forms of language that distinguishes us from other animals. However, non-verbal communication also plays a powerful role in most interactive and some non-interactive settings. Indeed, it has been suggested that non-verbal elements account for over 80 per cent of the content or meaning that is conveyed in face-to-face interactions. In most situations, effective communication depends on the appropriate and simultaneous use of both verbal and non-verbal channels. This is so natural that, even on the telephone, people tend automatically to use all sorts of gestures that cannot be seen by the person on the other end of the line. Chapter 2 of this book looks at different types and modes of communication, drawing on state-of-the-art knowledge in social psychology and communication studies. It distinguishes between intrapersonal (i.e. within person) and interpersonal (i.e. between person) communication, with the former being used for such activities as reflection, problem solving and self-evaluation, whereas the latter involves interacting with others. The chapter moves on to discuss factors relating to communication between two people, and among small groups and with larger audiences. Finally, it briefly considers communication using computers and other forms of advanced technology. These latter topics are covered more fully in Chapter 7.

A number of theories and models have been put forward to explain the way in which we communicate. Chapter 3 outlines the three main theoretical approaches within communication studies; namely, the process approach, semiotic analysis and cultural studies. It also covers other relevant models and approaches, such as Transactional Analysis, and models of health behaviour (the Health Belief Model and Theory of Planned Behaviour) and health communication. Finally, given that in many instances health communications involve trying to persuade a person or people to take a recommended course of action, the chapter overviews the two main theories of persuasion (the Elaboration Likelihood and Heuristic Systematic models). In each case, the key concepts underlying the various approaches, models and theories will be introduced and evaluated by drawing on empirical evidence, where this exists.

Communication between different 'players' in the healthcare process

In order to maximize the chances of effective communication, it is not only necessary to understand the relevant theoretical background, but it is also important to take account of current research in the area. Any attempts to improve communication practice must be grounded in sound empirical evidence. Chapter 4 reviews such evidence in relation to interactions between the different 'players' in the healthcare process, including healthcare providers, patients, family, friends, carers, and so on.

Many of the empirical studies that have examined the effects of communication skills on patient satisfaction and health behaviours and outcomes have involved looking at interactions between individual healthcare providers (most notably doctors) and individual patients. Accordingly, Chapter 4 reviews much of the recent research on health professional–patient communication. It looks at why effective communication is important, and what factors contribute to 'good' communication, as well as to 'poor' communication. It approaches the topic from the perspective of both health professionals and patients. The chapter also considers particular 'patient communication' issues that may arise for those working in health professions, such as nursing and pharmacy, who are now taking on new extended roles (such as extended and supplementary drug prescribing).

The importance of communication extends beyond these healthcare provider–patient relationships. Effective communication is also necessary in interactions between different healthcare providers, between health service administrators and patients, between healthcare providers and carers or family members, between patients and family members, and so on. Chapter 4 also considers the role that communication plays in some of these other relationships. Finally, it looks at communication in small group settings, such as case meetings.

Communicating with particular audiences and in difficult circumstances

Clearly, the same type of communication skills and behaviours will not be best suited to all types of interaction and in all settings. Interacting with certain types of patient and interested parties may require particular skills and raise particular challenges. Chapter 5 considers some of the issues raised when communicating with particular audiences, including older people, children and adolescents, those with low IQ or other forms of mental impairment, parents and other carers, and different ethnic groups, as well as with those termed 'uncommunicative' people.

In addition to having to communicate with these different audiences, the need to communicate certain types of information can create particular challenges. Chapter 6 begins by looking at some of the issues raised when trying to communicate information about risk and uncertainty, which is central to many healthcare interactions, and has been shown to be a particular challenge. Discussion of risk and uncertainty is often central to healthcare settings such as genetic counselling, where critical decisions may need to be made and ongoing counselling may be required. One relatively common, and particularly difficult, form of information that has to be imparted in healthcare settings is 'bad news'. This can cover a whole range of stressful situations, such as having to tell a patient that they have a terminal illness, or having to inform close relatives of a patient's unexpected death. The chapter therefore also deals with many of the challenges raised by having to communicate such 'bad news'. Finally, Chapter 6 considers many of the important ethical issues that are raised by these demanding circumstances.

Communication on a wider scale

The importance of effective communication is not just relevant to inter-actions that relate to patients in healthcare settings, such as general prac-titioner (GP) practices, hospitals and clinics, but is also fundamental at the wider public health level. Indeed, it has been argued that the most significant determinant of health is social and economic circumstance, and that the least important is individual health behaviour (e.g. French and Adams, 2002). Thus, it is suggested that we should be focusing more effort on broader public health education campaigns than on trying to influence behaviour at the individual level, as the former is likely to be the most cost-effective approach to health promotion (Bennett and Murphy, 1997). Chapter 7 focuses on communicating with the wider public in order to promote better health. It considers the different approaches and strategies that have been taken, and evaluates their effectiveness. Following this, it looks at a number of the communication channels that have been used to disseminate informa-tion to the wider public. Over the past 20 years we have seen a vast increase in the number and availability of written Patient Information Leaflets. The chapter therefore assesses the development and effectiveness of this method of disseminating health information to the public. Another way of reaching mass audiences is to use the media, Internet and other modes of communi-cation. Again, in recent years, there has been a dramatic increase in the use of these channels to spread health-related information. However, such com-munication channels are often used by 'non-official sources' to disseminate health information, and the reliability of some of this has been called into question. Given the massive explosion in the public's engagement with such media to access health-related information, the chapter also considers the benefits and disadvantages of communication via these channels.

Improving communication skills

The possession of good communication or social skills pays more dividends in people's lives (Segrin and Flora, 2000, p. 490). Those with higher levels of skill have been found to cope more readily with stress, to adapt and adjust better to major life transitions and to be less likely to suffer from depression, loneliness or anxiety (Hargie and Dickson, 2004). In healthcare, the import-ance of health professionals having good communication skills is being increasingly recognized. Di Blasi et al. (2001) carried out a large systematic review across a number of countries and found that good practitioners' interpersonal skills made a significant difference to patients' well-being. They concluded that 'practitioners who attempted to form a warm and friendly relationship with their patients and reassured them that they would soon be better, were found to be more effective than practitioners who kept their consultations impersonal, formal or uncertain' (p. 760).

In the UK, the Health Services Commissioner's Annual Report (1993) identified poor or inadequate communication between patients and health professionals as the source of the majority of grievances that it dealt with. The Report went on to state that a major cause of the problems was inadequate training. Similarly, the International Medical Benefit/Risk Foundation (1993) concluded that 'insufficient attention has been given to the training of communication skills of healthcare professionals, and retuning these skills in continuing education programmes' (p. 14). Thus, a significant advance in the field of health communication has been the growing realization and acknowledgement that effective communication can be taught and learned. This realization led to the inclusion of communication skills as a key recommendation in the UK General Medical Council's guidance for medical schools, *Tomorrow's Doctors* (GMC, 1993). Unfortunately, however, the teaching of communication skills has largely remained outside the mainstream of clinical practice rather than being a fully integrated component (e.g. Hargie et al., 1998). This has led some medical students to undervalue the importance of this part of their training. The final chapter of this book focuses on how to improve communication skills by what is known as communication skills training. It reviews current empirical research in this area, and provides some practical guidelines and advice for health professionals in relation to such things as asking questions, listening effectively, and responding and providing feedback, particularly when faced with difficult or challenging circumstances such as those considered in Chapter 6.

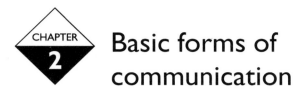

Basic forms of communication

Like all human communication, health communication can take different forms and occur in different contexts. A basic distinction in all human communication is between verbal (language-based) and non-verbal communication. Each of these can take place at a number of different levels, however. In terms of verbal communication, we can communicate within ourselves (intrapersonal communication) or with others (interpersonal communication). In the latter case, this can be done orally or via some other medium such as written language or signage. Interpersonal communication is frequently carried out between two people or in a small group. Such communications are usually transactional in nature, in that the individuals involved both affect, and are affected by, each other's contribution. However, in addition to these one-to-one or small-group interactions, we also need to engage in 'mass communication', for example in relation to health promotion and public health campaigns. This form of communication may involve different processes and raise additional issues. These are discussed more fully in Chapter 7.

Intrapersonal communication

Before looking at communication between two or more people (interpersonal communication) it is important to consider communication that occurs solely within ourselves. Intrapersonal communication is not only important for processes such as self-reflection and evaluation, but is also a key element that underlies our interactions with others. Thus, for example, two people will not necessarily interpret a statement made by the speaker or by a third person in the same way. Their interpretations will depend on their own particular decoding of the statement in the light of their prior knowledge and experience. Thus, Humpty Dumpty was clearly wrong in Lewis

Carroll's *Through the Looking Glass* when he insisted that 'when I use a word it means just what I choose it to mean' (Chrystal, 2005, p. 49). The fact that different people may interpret words and longer phrases in different ways can, on occasion, lead to misunderstanding and to unsuccessful interactions.

Intrapersonal communication may be a solely internal activity, where we reflect on a possible source of action or evaluate the consequences of what we have done, or it may involve some external expression, such as when we talk to ourselves or write for ourselves (such as making reminder notes or keeping a diary). According to Burton and Dimbleby (1995), there are four main elements of intrapersonal communication; namely, the core of self, needs and motivations, cognitions and monitoring the reactions of others.

The core of self

This is basically concerned with how we see and value ourselves; our self–image and personality. Our self-image not only depends on how we see and categorize ourselves, but also, importantly, on how we believe we are seen and categorized by others. As noted by Murray et al. (1996), the formation of self is not an independent event generated by an autonomous actor; rather it emerges through social interaction. Our self–image is said to be composed of physical attributes (e.g. our body image), intellectual attributes (e.g. how able or clever we think we are), and social or emotional attributes (e.g. how placid or emotional we believe we are). These attributes all contribute to our self–esteem; how we value ourselves. While our self-esteem is a major element of intrapersonal communication, it also affects how we communi-cate with others. People with high self-esteem, for example, have been noted to talk more firmly and confidently, whereas those with low esteem are more cautious. Similar differences have been observed in non–verbal behaviours, with those with high self-esteem being more open and ani-mated, using more expressive gestures.

Clearly, our self-image is not a static thing. We may change our image as a result of a significant change of situation or as a result of communications from others, particularly significant others and role models. However, self–images do tend to be relatively stable; other events and communications will only affect our self-image to the extent that we permit. As Gergen and Gergen (1988) noted, we often employ various self-maintenance strategies, such as selective or biased processing, or discrediting the 'communication source', in order retain our core self-image.

Needs and motivations

The second element involves the needs and motivations which drive the self to generate communications or interpret communications, and to change the way it presents itself in different sorts of interaction. According to

Burton and Dimbleby (1995), there are reasons why we choose to initiate thought processes or interact with others. For example, we are motivated to keep checking whether or not our view of ourselves 'holds true' in the light of communications from others. We are also motivated to construct an 'expression of self' that is appealing to others. Such needs and motivations may not always be explicit. They may drive our behaviour in a more subtle and unconscious way.

Cognitions

The third element of intrapersonal communication outlined by Burton and Dimbleby (1995) is cognition: the internal activities by which we make sense of the world. The way in which we generate and interpret communications will depend on our prior knowledge, experiences and values that we hold. According to Burton and Dimbleby, there are five main cognitive processes involved in intrapersonal processing. These are decoding (i.e. interpreting communications from others), integration (i.e. relating these to other information), memory (i.e. remembering the information), schemata (i.e. ways of organizing information) and encoding (i.e. composing communications to transmit to others). Each of these will be affected by our past knowledge and experience, as well as by particular beliefs and emotional factors.

Monitoring the reactions of others

The final element of intrapersonal communication, according to Burton and Dimbleby (1995), involves the internal activity of monitoring the reactions of others to our communications. We constantly obtain and check reactions from others in order to see what effect we are having on them, and to adjust future behaviour if appropriate. This involves monitoring both their verbal and non-verbal behaviours. The latter often provides a particularly influential source of feedback, as non-verbal communication tends to be more automatic and less open to control by others. As we will see later in this chapter, people may say one thing verbally but their body language or facial expression may portray a different picture (a phenomenon known as 'social leakage').

Interpersonal communication

The study of interpersonal communication has a long history. As noted by Hargie and Dickson (2004), the oldest essay ever discovered (written about 3000 BC) consisted of advice on speaking effectively in public. The most common type of interpersonal communication is face-to-face interaction between two or more people. Such interactions typically comprise a sequence of events and behaviours. Brooks and Heath (1993, p. 3) defined interpersonal communication as 'the process by which information, meanings, and feelings are shared by persons through the exchange of verbal and non-verbal messages'. Hargie and Dickson (2004), elaborated on this by stating that communication is essentially a process that consists of the following main elements:

1 Two or more communicators (i.e. a source and a receiver).
2 A message (the content of the communication).
3 The medium or the particular means of conveying the message, with the three main types being presentational (e.g. voice, body), representational (e.g. books, photos) and technological (e.g. television). The first is pivotal in interpersonal communication.
4 The channel (i.e. what connects the communicators and accommodates the medium; e.g. vocal–auditory, gestural–visual).
5 A code (i.e. system of meaning shared by a group, such as the English language).
6 Noise (this is not just mere sounds but includes any interference with the success of the communicative act).
7 Feedback.
8 The context in which the interaction occurs.

Communication can be a one-way or two-way process. In the former case, for example, a directive might be issued or a statement or speech given, with no opportunity for response from the recipient. This type of communication is reflected in Theodorson and Theodorson's (1969) definition of communication as the transmission of information, ideas, attitudes or emotion from one person or group to another (or others), primarily through symbols. In contrast, two-way communication involves interaction, with the different parties being able to contribute to and control the flow of events. The key elements in such a process are mutuality and shared perceptions and understandings. This type of communication is reflected in Rogers and Kincaid's later definition of communication as 'a process in which the participants create and share information with one another in order to reach a mutual understanding' (1981, p. 63).

The one-way, two-way distinction is relevant to considerations of 'power'. Typically, in one-way communication, the sender is perceived to have all the power and control, whereas in two-way interactions there is typically a more balanced power relationship. However, as Windahl and Signitzer (1992) noted, this is not necessarily the case, as the two-way process can be designed in such a way as to give only the illusion of influence and power. Many two-way interactions that occur in health settings involve unbalanced power relationships, with senior doctors in particular dominating interactions and being seen to be less open to challenge.

As noted earlier, and in Chapter 1, however, much interpersonal communication is a genuine two-way process; it is frequently transactional in nature in that the people involved both influence and are influenced by the other participants. They each bring different prior experiences, values and 'personalities' that will influence the interaction, as will the social context in which it occurs. As far as the latter is concerned, people usually interact differently in formal settings, such as meetings, from how they converse with each other in social gatherings, such as parties. Participants in the interaction will also have different motivations and needs, that will influence the transactional nature of the process. Researchers have studied this aspect of interaction, using a tool called 'Transactional Analysis'; this will be covered in the next chapter.

Interpersonal communication can be thought of as a skill. Hargie (1997, p. 12) defined interpersonal skill as the 'process whereby the individual implements a set of goal directed, inter-related situationally appropriate social behaviours which are learned and controlled'. As outlined by Hargie and Dickson (2004), this encompasses seven components of skill:

1 Skilled performance is a process which involves formulating goals and action plans, implementing these plans, monitoring the effects of behaviour, adjusting and abandoning goals and responses in the light of outcomes, and taking cognizance of other people and the context in which the interaction occurs.
2 Skilled behaviours are goal directed, although goals are not always conscious.
3 Skilled behaviours must be inter related in that they are synchronized to achieve a goal.
4 Skills should be appropriate to the situation in which they are used.
5 Skills are defined in terms of identifiable units of behaviour. Skill is reflected in the performance of communicative behaviours.
6 Skilled behaviours are learned and developed through a number of stages.
7 Skills should be under the cognitive control of the individual.

Verbal language

Although we can convey our intended meanings in many different ways (e.g. speech, body communication, hand signals), it is usually our verbal language (particularly the spoken aspects) that is considered to be primary. The use of spoken and written language is a key factor in what distinguishes us from other animals. The capacity for spoken language and symbol manipulation arose between about 2 million and 300 000 years ago as *Homo sapiens* became differentiated from other species. Verbal language is so pervasive that it has been noted that every human group that has been studied by anthropologists has a lexicon (i.e. an internal dictionary of meanings) and a grammar (a way of organizing those meanings).

We use verbal language for many different things. Thus, it is used to generate meanings, to express ideas and feelings, and for interacting with and controlling others. It is also central to the intrapersonal communication processes of thinking and reflection. Language is voluntary, in that it is under our control. Most of us do not automatically generate words without any conscious awareness of what we are saying and why. Verbal language is also symbolic, in that it represents something other than itself, as well as being systematic, in that it is not made up of random strings of symbols. It primarily operates in two different modalities – speech and writing – with speech being regarded as primary.

Speech and writing

Verbal language can be spoken or written. Generally, speech is a more spontaneous process, whereas writing tends to be more deliberate. The result of this is that speech is often less precise than writing and more loosely structured syntactically. An interesting exception to this is the use of email and text messaging which tends to be much more like spoken than formal written language. People are more likely to use colloquialisms and ungrammatical phrases when communicating via such media. In addition, speech takes place in real time, whereas writing is less time constrained and can be reviewed. Speech is also connected, in that phonemes (the basic units of sound) blend into each other, whereas writing uses discrete units (letters).

Humans have been speaking for many tens of thousands of years, and may have been signing for much longer. But writing is a more recent development. The first true writing system is said to have been invented by the Sumarians (now in Iraq) around 5000 years ago. Even after writing was invented, however, it failed to have a major impact on the world. Only a small minority of languages were coded into written form and, even today, it is still the case that the majority of the languages used across the world do not have writing systems associated with them. Furthermore, until probably the twentieth century, only a relatively small proportion of the population was literate (i.e. could read and write). It is now estimated that more than half of the world population can read and write at least one language, although this is not necessarily their native language. The fact that the process of becoming literate involves considerable work has meant that people have tended to be reluctant to change the written form of languages. So while speech is constantly changing and evolving, many of these changes have not been reflected in the associated writing systems. This has resulted in writing becoming more conservative and 'old fashioned' compared with speech. It has often been noted, for example, that travellers who have learned a foreign language at school, mostly through reading and writing, have been surprised by how little they can understand of what the local people say when they visit the country where the language is spoken.

Non-verbal communication

Non-verbal communication can be thought of as all forms of direct communication not exclusively relying on the use of written or spoken words (Hargie and Dickson, 2004). The vast majority of interpersonal communications comprise both verbal and non-verbal components. Although the verbal component of interactions is clearly important, research has shown that the non-verbal elements can account for up to 80 per cent of the content or meaning that is conveyed in face-to-face interactions. Speech rarely occurs in isolation from non-verbal cues. In most everyday social situations, verbal and non-verbal behaviours are complexly intertwined, each to varying degrees defining the other in the process of conveying meaning. As several researchers have commented, we speak with our vocal organs but we converse with our whole body.

People can produce around 700 000 different facial expressions, physical gestures, and movements. Even the briefest interaction can involve the fleeting and simultaneous use of a large number of these communication devices (Fraser and Burcell, 2001). Furthermore, the non-verbal components can be thought of as being primary in that they are less subject to control. When there is a mismatch between the verbal and non-verbal messages being conveyed (a phenomenon known as 'social leakage'), it is likely that the non-verbal component is conveying the 'truer message'. Taking account of this, Burton and Dimbleby (1995) proposed that we need to distinguish between linguistic competence (our ability to use verbal language) and our communicative competence (our ability to use forms of verbal and non-verbal language in ways that are appropriate to the situation).

Relating successfully to other people requires the ability to display appropriate non-verbal behaviours, but also to be sensitive to the non-verbal communications of others. Northouse and Northouse (1998) proposed that non-verbal communication has special relevance in healthcare, primarily because patients pay close attention to the non-verbal signals of health professionals, and may rely on these to give a rapid means of gaining information before any verbal interaction takes place. Similarly, doctors and other health professionals should pay close attention to patients' non-verbal signals, particularly where there is a mismatch between these and what the patient is saying. In recognition of factors such as this, communication skills training now routinely covers these important non-verbal, as well as verbal, aspects of communication (see Chapter 8). This is crucial as studies such as Rosenblum et al. (1994) have shown that it is possible to predict grades assigned to medical students by clinical supervisors by rating a sample of the students' non-verbal behaviour while interacting with patients.

Non-verbal communication has been noted to perform a number of different functions in social interactions:

1 To replace verbal communication in situations where it may be impossible or inappropriate to talk.

2 To support and validate our verbal messages. Thus, facial expressions and gestures should reinforce what is being said, rather than conveying a different message.
3 To communicate our feelings and emotions (such as anger, fear, happiness).
4 To regulate interactions and provide feedback. Non-verbal signals, such as shifts in posture and raised eyebrows, can be used to initiate and terminate interactions and to regulate the flow of messages.
5 To negotiate relationships in respect of factors such as dominance and control.
6 For self-presentation and maintenance of self-image, for example by choice of clothes, hairstyle and so on.

Non-verbal communication is traditionally divided into six different elements.

Kinesics

This is often referred to as 'body language'. It includes our posture and body movements, such as those of the hands, arms, feet, head and eyes, that contribute to our gestures and facial expressions. These all provide powerful communication signals. Gaze, for example, has been noted to play a role in monitoring and regulating interactions and expressing our feelings and emotions, and has been said to be the most information-rich and important of the non-verbal communication channels (Kleinke, 1986). The amount and pattern of gazing can provide information about people's attentiveness, feelings, credibility, honesty, competence and relative status. In a similar way, facial expressions are a powerful signal of our emotions. It has been shown that basic emotions such as happiness, surprise, sadness, fear, anger and disgust are associated with quite distinctive patterns of facial expression (Ekman, 1982) and that these are relatively universal. For example, we all tend to raise our eyebrows when we express surprise, whereas we do the opposite when we display anger or disgust (see Figure 2.1). In contrast, the use of gesture varies much more according to culture and the situation. Italians, for instance, use hand gestures to a much greater extent than the British. Ekman and Friesen (1969) identified six main types of gesture:

1 Emblems (signs that are often used to replace speech)
2 Illustrators (that accompany speech to clarify it)
3 Regulators (to orchestrate conversation and ensure smooth turn taking)
4 Affect displays (hands, for example, can be used to show embarrassment, nervousness, aggression or shame)
5 Adaptors (often used to release self-tension)
6 Head nods (which can either replace or complement speech).

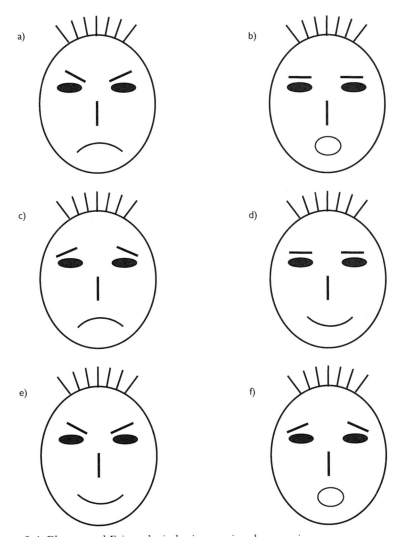

Figure 2.1 Ekman and Friesen's six basic emotional expressions

Note: a = anger, b = fear, c = sadness, d = happiness, e = surprise, f = disgust

Paralinguistics

This includes all our sound patterns that are content-free. It refers to vocal sounds, such as 'ah-ha' and 'um', which often are integrated with our words. It also includes the way words are spoken (e.g. in terms of intensity and pitch) and features such as pauses and speed of speech. Each person's voice is unique in terms of how it varies on these different dimensions, and these paralinguistic aspects vary depending on the particular message that is being conveyed, either intentionally or otherwise. Knapp and Hall (1997) reviewed evidence showing that the use of paralanguage influences judgements about speakers (e.g. their personality and emotional state), the presentation of the message (in terms of excitement or competence), and how the message should be received (e.g. in a tongue-in-cheek, sober, or respectful way).

Proxemics

This refers largely to personal space and the distance between people, and how we make use of it. In terms of the distance between people, Hall (1996) identified four different 'distance zones' (intimate, personal, social and public). In western cultures, intimate distance tends to be about 1.5 feet, personal distance is between this and 2.5 feet, and social distance is between 4 and 12 feet (Northouse and Northouse, 1998). These distances have been noted to vary for people from other cultures (as do several other aspects of non-verbal communication). It is interesting that when people become patients their ideal personal space is often 'invaded', and this may lead to feelings of loss of dignity and increased helplessness. Wherever possible, health professionals should be aware of this and try to give attention to patients' privacy needs.

Physical contact, such as touch

Touch can take different forms and convey different messages. How it is interpreted will depend on the context and the relationship between the people involved. It has been noted that the extent to which touch is used is affected by a number of factors, including cultural background and gender. In general, men touch women more often than women touch men, and people are more likely to touch members of the opposite sex (Henley, 1973). Jones and Yarbrough (1985) identified five discrete categories of touch:

1 Positive affect (e.g. to show appreciation)
2 Playful (e.g. to show humour)
3 Control (e.g. to draw attention)
4 Ritualistic (e.g. greetings)
5 Task related (e.g. a nurse taking a pulse).

Touch is clearly important in many healthcare settings, but health professionals need to be careful when touching patients. In some contexts, it may be appropriate to ask the patient's permission before touching them. Whenever touch is used, it is important to be aware of the patient's response. In support of this, Hollinger and Buschmann (1993) found that, when hospitalized, older adults' perception of touch was said to be most positive when it was appropriate to the situation, did not impose a greater level of intimacy than desired, was not condescending and did not detract from their sense of independence and autonomy.

Environmental characteristics

These refer to the physical setting in which an interaction occurs, such as whether it is indoors or outside, the type, layout and decoration of rooms and so on. Noise levels and types of sound are also important. These environmental factors can reflect on the person inhabiting the space and can shape interpersonal contact. It has been shown that the physical setting can influence our mood, how we view a social situation, our judgements of others and the form an interaction will take. Clearly, different types of setting are appropriate for different types of interaction, and it is important to ensure that a room's layout and so on will facilitate rather than impede effective communication. As we will see in Chapter 8, communication skills training now routinely covers advice about appropriate settings (such as room layout) for consultations, rather than just focusing on what is being said (and how).

Personal characteristics and adornments

Personal characteristics that play a role in non-verbal communication include our body shape, skin colour and facial features. Additional signals are given by our clothing, jewellery and hairstyle. Some of these features (such as hairstyle or what we wear) are subject to our control, whereas others (such as our skin colour or our facial features) are not. Studies have shown that there are powerful effects of appearance on judgements of intelligence, warmth, friendliness and social confidence (Smith and Mackie, 2000). Unfortunately, the notion of the 'dumb blonde' is not a fallacy, in the sense that some people may actually take this view in the complete absence of any supporting evidence. Clearly, it is important for healthcare professionals to dress appropriately for the situation. One would not normally expect a doctor, for example, to break the news of diagnosis of a terminal illness or patient death wearing a casual T-shirt and shorts.

The use of language

The study of language has often focused on small units such as sounds, words and sentences. However, these are rarely used in isolation; rather, they are used to make up conversations, speeches, instructions, essays, and so on. These larger segments of language are usually structured according to par-ticular rules and traditions. Any single and coherent piece of language is referred to as a 'discourse'. Spoken languages such as English are based on the rule-governed structuring of basic sounds (phonemes) into units of meanings (morphemes). These are further structured by morphological and syntactical rules into words and sentences respectively. The meanings of these utterances are determined by semantic rules. Together, these rules make up the grammar of the language.

Language is used for many different purposes. Trask (1998), for example, identified eight different uses, which will all involve the subtle blend of both verbal and non-verbal elements:

1   To pass on information
2   To amuse ourselves
3   To entertain others
4   To express our individuality
5   To maintain and express our membership of a group
6   To persuade others to do something
7   To establish and maintain relationships with others
8   To express emotions.

Conversations

The most frequent use of language is to converse with others, and this is the kind of discourse that is most familiar to the majority of us. A conversation can be thought of as a connected exchange of remarks spoken by two or more people. Conversations have an array of complex rules that govern every phase of the interaction (Clark, 1985). The co-operative nature of conversation is fundamental. Thus, it is usually the case that only one person speaks at a time and that an individual's remarks usually relate to the preceding remark or remarks. Burton and Dimbleby (1995) identified seven different elements of conversation making, these being openings, turn taking, closure, questioning, listening, using non-verbal communication, and recognizing feedback. Non-verbal communication was covered earlier. We will now look briefly at each of the remainder.

Openings   The way people open a conversation can have a significant influence on, and set the tone for, the rest of the exchange. Greetings can be conceived of as structured formalized sequences through which we have a greater opportunity to make important points and to create an impact on others. The opening of a conversation can be done verbally (e.g. through standard greetings, such as 'good morning' or 'hello') and/or non-verbally (e.g. using eye contact, facial expression, touch, proximity, and so on). The way a conversation is opened will depend on the context, the relationship between the participants, and the purpose of the conversation. If the purpose is more formal, then touching, close proximity or a casual greeting might be inappropriate, whereas an opening such as 'good morning, I have arranged this discussion so that . . .' and a handshake may well be more suitable.

Turn taking   In most conversations, each person finishes speaking before another starts. This is facilitated by the fact that we use signals to indicate that we are about to finish speaking or that another person wishes to contribute something. Such signals include using intonation of the voice or eye contact or other gestures, or by asking an explicit question such as 'what do you think?' Listeners also use non-verbal communications, such as gestures and paralinguistics, as well as verbal ones, to signal that they would like to make a contribution to the conversation. They may, for example, make an utterance, such as 'um' or 'eh', or move closer, or use a hand gesture to indicate their desire to talk next.

Closure   The nature of the relationship, the context, and the preceding conversation will influence the way it is closed. In more formal interactions, a person might summarize what has been said and agreed. Similarly, attempts might be made to check the other person's understanding. Less formal conversations might end with a smile or hug, or a phrase such as 'bye' or 'see you later'. Non-verbal signals, such as breaking eye contact, standing up or straightening papers may also be used to effect closure. An ideal closure is where both participants leave the interaction feeling satisfied with it and happy to re-engage with each other when required.

Questioning   A question is any statement or non-verbal act that invites an answer (Stewart and Cash, 2000). Questions can be used to maintain and influence the course of interactions and to obtain specific pieces of information. To ask a question is one of the most powerful tools in communication (Hawkins and Power, 1999), as questions are at the heart of most interpersonal interactions. Clearly, question asking is an important factor in the work of many professionals. In healthcare settings, a common form of questioning is the medical interview. This will be covered more fully in Chapter 8.

There are two basic types of question. Open questions (such as 'how was your holiday?') encourage longer, unstructured answers, whereas closed questions (such as 'did you go to Paris this year?') often encourage simple yes/no answers. Healthcare professionals often use closed questions to shorten the length of consultations, but there is a danger that key information may be missed. Both open and closed questions can be phrased in a neutral or leading way. Leading questions tend to bias the response that is given, and should be used with caution (if at all). An example of a leading question might be a healthcare provider asking 'how much more pain are you feeling?', which assumes that the person is feeling more pain.

An analysis of the use of questions in doctor–patient communications has shown that doctors ask the majority of questions and patients provide most of the answers (e.g. Brashers et al., 2002). Furthermore, it has been noted that when patients do ask questions these are often marked by speech disturbance, indicating discomfort at requesting information from doctors (e.g. West, 1983). Similarly, Skelton and Hobbs (1999) noted that patient questions were often prefaced by phrases such as 'I was wondering . . .', whereas doctors rarely used such expressions. Interestingly, studies have also shown that in community settings, such as community pharmacies, the ratio of patient-to-doctor questions is much higher (e.g. Morrow et al., 1993), probably reflecting the perceived control differential between the questioner and respondent. Thus, in most situations, it is the person of higher status who asks most of the questions. As we will see in Chapter 8, a key component of communication skills training for patients involves encouraging them to ask more, and more effective, questions.

Recognizing feedback   Feedback is a fundamental aspect of communication. De Vito (1998) defined it as the message that is sent back to the speaker concerning reactions to what has been said. Thus, having acted, communicators need to rely on knowledge of their performance together with outcomes that may have accrued in order to reach decisions as to what to do next, and to alter subsequent responses accordingly. We clearly need to be aware of, and sensitive to, the feedback of other participants in a conversation. This is a key element of active listening, which is discussed more fully in Chapter 8. It is necessary for people to be sensitive to the particular choice of words in a conversation and to the accompanying non-verbal signals. As mentioned earlier, the latter usually provide powerful signals and may conflict with the verbal messages that are given out.

Communication in groups

Social groups occupy much of our day-to-day lives. Most of us work in groups, socialize or play in groups, and represent our attitudes and views through groups. Groups are a vital part of people's life spans (Heath and Bryant, 2000). They provide companionship, support, and even a sense of identity, as well as helping us to perform our jobs effectively. Interestingly, it has been noted that in healthcare settings, many functions that were once provided by an individual are now team based, and that groups are being used more and more among health professionals in both acute care and community settings (Northouse and Northouse, 1998).

In general, a group refers to a collection of people who interact in some way and share common goals or interests. As noted by Douglas (2000), any collection of people who are aware of each other's presence could be called a group. However, what really distinguishes a group from such a collection of people is that in a group there is some form of interdependence between members. Thus, Johnson and Johnson defined a group as

two or more individuals in face-to-face interaction, each aware of his or her membership in the group, each aware of their membership in the group, each aware of others who belong to the group, and each aware of their positive interdependence as they strive to achieve mutual goals.

(1987, p. 8)

A group can vary in size from a relatively small number, such as a committee or medical care team, to a very large number, such as an ethnic or professional group. Although the Johnson and Johnson definition accurately characterizes many groups, such as family, friendship, work and support groups, it is less appropriate when applied to larger collections of people (such as ethnic groups) or to groups who primarily communicate in other ways (e.g. computer-mediated communication groups). It is usually the case that membership of a group signals certain things, and people are frequently categorized or stereotyped according to such membership. This applies not only to large ethnic or professional groups, but also to smaller work, family and social groups.

Small-group communication refers to the verbal and non-verbal communication that occurs among a collection of individuals whose relationships make them, to some degree, interdependent (Northouse and Northouse, 1998). Intra-group communication is a necessary prerequisite for the emergence and perpetuation of norms and roles, as well as for conformity and coherence and the achievement of desired outcomes (Hargie and Dickson, 2004). As several researchers have noted, groups emerge through communication and it is in this way that they achieve their objectives. At the same time, the communication process is heavily influenced in turn by the internal structures that are created. Similarly, Brilhart and Galanes (1998, p. 44) argued that communication is the verbal and non-verbal process by which individuals forge themselves into a group, maintain the group and co-ordinate their effort.

Small-group communication involves many similar processes to interactions between two people, but will also involve some different ones. In one-to-one interactions, the way we present ourselves depends on our perception of the other participant and the social context. In a group situation, we become more aware of playing a role in relation to the group. This may, for example, be a leadership role or a more subordinate role. Similarly, it may be a 'challenger' role or a 'pacifier' role. In addition, we are constrained by our perception of the group, its members and purpose. Although our participation in all interactions is affected by our needs and motivations, in group interactions it is more likely that these may need to be modified or subordinated in order to facilitate the effective functioning of the group. Our behaviours will also depend on the dynamics of the group and degree of group cohesion.

The relationships and processes of a group are rarely static. During the course of their development, most groups start to operate according to certain 'rules', standards and boundaries that govern the group's interactions, although these are often not stated explicitly. The emergence of such norms is of crucial importance in regulating the activities of group members. Norms can be defined as those behaviours, attitudes and perceptions that are approved of by the group and expected of its members (Hargie and Dickson, 2004). Norms may, for example, cover the degree of formality of the group, which topics can be openly discussed and which should not, and how much emotion can be expressed. Group pressure tends to enforce and reinforce these standards and boundaries so that members' behaviour and communications are brought in line with one another. This usually results in the group becoming more cohesive with time, so that the members' shared experiences and increased familiarity with each other contribute to effective working relationships. Group norms serve a function for the individual, in that they specify the range of behaviour that is acceptable and appropriate for the situation. However, they also serve functions for the group, in that they co-ordinate the actions of members towards the fulfilment of group goals. In general, the more co-operative a group, the more freely communication will flow. Members will share and show interest in others' ideas, gaining from as well as contributing to the group's interactions. In contrast, competitiveness between members can seriously impede the effective functioning of a group, in that it can lead to people becoming inhibited or deliberately holding back relevant information.

Whereas norms tend to apply to all group members, clearly these members will not all act alike, and they will usually take different roles which may emerge with time. Bormann (1990) defined role in a small group as that set of perceptions and expectations shown by members about the behaviour of an individual in both the task and social dimension of group interaction. Studies that have analysed interactions between group members have shown that some members typically participate more in discussions than others. This is often a function of the status of the person, their knowledge and personality, as well as the group size. It has also been noted that while high contributors tend to provide information, give opinions and make suggestions, low contributors (when they do participate) tend to ask more questions or express agreement.

The effective functioning of a group will clearly depend on the quality of the verbal and non-verbal communication that takes place within the group. Speaking and listening must be co-ordinated with several other people, rather than just one other. Similarly, group members need to be aware of the needs and feelings of several other people and take account of them when making their own contributions. Generally, in group settings, one has to be more sensitive to what one is saying and how it is being said, so as not to offend other group members. However, it is more difficult to monitor the verbal and non-verbal reactions of several people, as opposed to just one. Clearly, conflicts can arise, and these can occur for a number of reasons. For example, group members may have competing aims or needs, or there may be a clash in relation to the role they expect themselves or others to play. Whatever the cause, conflict can be managed in a number of different ways, with the three most prominent being avoidance, diffusion and confrontation. Conflict management and resolution are covered more fully in Chapter 8.

Mass communication

In addition to one-to-one and small-group interactions, communications can also be conveyed to wider segments of the population. In terms of health-related information, much of this communication falls under the umbrella of health promotion or public health campaigns. Mass communication can occur through a number of different media. These include written leaflets and brochures, advertising hoardings and posters, newspapers, magazines, radio, television, computer systems and the Internet.

Mass communication is typically a one-way process, with the message going from sender to receiver. However, the increasing use of computers to disseminate health information has allowed for some degree of interactivity, such as that embodied in many computerized health information systems, where the information that is given to users will depend on personal details that they have entered. Clearly, the success of any mass communication campaign will depend on the message reaching the target audience and being interpreted and applied appropriately. In most cases, the aim will be to change behaviour, for example, encouraging people to stop smoking, practise safe sex, eat more healthily, and so on. Mass communication raises a number of challenges, such as identifying and reaching the right audience, and ensuring that the message is appropriate for that audience and is likely to be acted on. The different forms of mass communication, and some of the issues raised, are discussed more fully in Chapter 7, where we look at health promotion and communicating with the wider public.

Summary

The present chapter has distinguished between intrapersonal and interpersonal communication, and has outlined the basic concepts and processes involved in each. It has looked at interactions between two individuals and in small groups, as well as the topic of mass communication. The next chapter looks at some of the underlying theoretical approaches that have been put forward to explain how and why we communicate in particular ways.

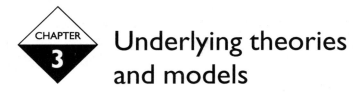

Underlying theories and models

The previous chapter considered different types and modes of communication. The current chapter moves on to look at some of the underlying theories and models that have been put forward to account for how we communicate, as well as what governs our health behaviours and how we persuade other people to change their behaviours. We begin by looking at the three main approaches to the study of communication outlined by Burton and Dimbleby (1995): the process, the semiotic and the cultural studies approach. We then consider what is now a classic, and is probably the best known, model of communication – the Shannon-Weaver (1949) model – as an early example of the processing approach. We also look at the more recent model of interpersonal communication that has been developed by Hargie and colleagues (e.g. Hargie, 1997). As the book is specifically about health communication, we next review two well-known models of health behaviour: the Health Belief Model (Rosenstock, 1974) and the Theory of Planned Behaviour (Azjen, 1988). Elements from both communication theories and models of health behaviours are brought together in Northouse and Northouse's (1998) model of health communication, which we consider next. A central element in the Northouse and Northouse model is the idea of transactions. These transactions can be studied using Berne's (e.g. 1958) Transactional Analysis. This methodological approach helps us to explain why we communicate in particular ways, how we carry out the communication and what affects the course of it. A brief overview is provided here. Finally, given that a key aim of many health communications is to persuade people to change their behaviour, we look at the two main theories of persuasion (the Elaboration Likelihood Model and the Heuristic Systematic Model).

The Process, Semiotic and Cultural Studies approaches to communication

Burton and Dimbleby (1995) identified and outlined three different approaches to understanding and explaining communication. These are the Process, Semiotic, and Cultural Studies approach. Although we describe each separately, they do have elements in common, and most communications can be accounted for using a combination of two or more approaches.

The Process approach

This is probably the most dominant of the three approaches. The Process approach basically describes what is happening when we communicate, how it happens, and what it is affected by. As is evident from its name, this approach focuses on the key processes involved in any communication, such as the encoding and decoding of messages, and the transmission of signs and intended meanings. It is about communication as action which influences the behaviour of others and produces change. Communication is seen as being active, dynamic, continuous and irreversible, and as taking place within a social and physical context. It takes account of, and shifts, according to needs, the audience and the given situation. When the communication involves two or more people, verbal and non-verbal signs are used to convey meaning and to negotiate different kinds of relationship. The processes involved include recognition, understanding and evaluation of others, and using feedback from them to alter our subsequent behaviours. Social skills involve controlling the flow of signs so that their meanings are acceptable to those involved. Group communications involve additional processes, such as role playing and bonding, and patterns of decision making.

The Semiotic approach

The second approach outlined by Burton and Dimbleby focuses more on the particular signs that are used in the communication process and the meanings that are generated by these signs. The approach is also concerned with the underlying structure of communications. Not surprisingly, the Semiotic approach has its roots in classical language study, and encompasses both semantic and syntactic aspects of language. The notion of codes and structures within a code provide a means of analysing communications. Thus, semiotics is concerned with the internal production of meaning from external signs recognized in communicative activity. Within this approach, social interaction can be seen as an exchange of signs between people and as being bound by conventions, so that we select particular signs that are appropriate to particular situations. Perception of others is about recognizing the signs of communication for what they are, and then making sense of them. Similarly, self-presentation is about the conscious selection of particular signs for particular effect.

The Cultural Studies approach

The final approach outlined by Burton and Dimbleby has a fair amount in common with the Semiotic approach. Like semiotics, Cultural Studies is concerned with signs and meanings, but in relation to particular social groupings within society. The approach is also interested in the divisions between social groupings and in the naturalization of these divisions through the force of ideology working within the social system. Craig (1999) defined it as 'a symbolic process that produces and reproduces shared sociocultural patterns' (p. 119). That is, it is the shared system of beliefs, values, language, political economy and other institutional arrangements that make communication possible. Overall, then, the approach is concerned with the creation of a distinctive culture through communication, and how culture can be maintained and transmitted through our communications. In turn, communication is seen primarily as an instrument of identity or power and even repression. Our perception of others tends to endorse social divisions and power relations. Self-presentation includes statements about social position and social attitudes. In terms of group communication, the approach is concerned with what the communication of the group signifies for group identity, the group's relationship with the rest of society, and the ways in which its social position is made natural and acceptable.

The Shannon-Weaver model of communication

The Shannon-Weaver (1949) model is an early example of models developed according to a processing or, more specifically, an information-processing approach. According to the model, information is selected by an 'information source' and this is then encoded into a message (see Figure 3.1). The message is then transmitted via a signal, through a channel (such as speech) to a receiver. The receiver decodes (that is, interprets) the signal and acts on it, for example, by passing the message on to some destination. The other concept identified in the Shannon-Weaver model is 'noise source'. During the course of its transmission, the message can be disturbed by factors, such as audible sounds or distortions, that may change the meaning of the message. Thus, in this way, the model outlines the flow of information from source to destination. However, despite being recognized as a 'classic' communication model, it is generally acknowledged to be limited, as the message is basically seen to flow in one direction – from source to receiver. The model does not easily allow for the transactional (two-way) nature of communications.

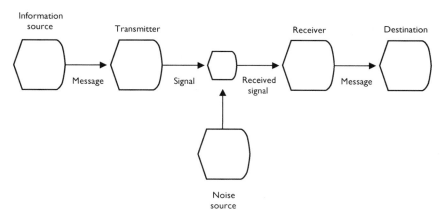

Figure 3.1 Shannon–Weaver model of communication

Hargie and colleagues' model of interpersonal communication

More recent communication models have taken a less simplistic view of interactions. Hargie and colleagues (e.g. Dickson et al., 1997; Hargie, 1997; Hargie and Marshall, 1986), for example, have put forward a model of interpersonal communication (see Figure 3.2) that rests on three basic assumptions. These are that people act purposefully, they are sensitive to the effects of their actions and they take steps to modify subsequent actions in the light of this information. It is stressed that, due to the dynamic and changing character of communication, both participants are, one and the same time, senders and receivers of information. The model identifies six basic elements of skilled interpersonal interaction (the person–situation context, goals, mediating processes, responses, feedback and perceptions). Hargie and colleagues argue that what takes place when people engage in communication is partly a feature of the particular attributes and characteristics of the individual (including their knowledge, values, emotions, motives, attitudes and expectations, as well as such factors as age and gender), and partly due to the parameters of the shared situation in which the interaction occurs, including the role demands placed on participants. It is also recognized that as well as being affected by physical context, role demands and so on, interactions are also influenced by culture. Intercultural differences extend much further than just differences in verbal language. They also encompass differences in non–verbal communication, as well as the underlying social order and the meanings of values that give it form. Thus, cultural influences permeate values, beliefs and practices, and govern how people conduct themselves in interaction with others.

Other key elements in the model include goals (i.e. the desired end states towards which people strive; Berger, 1995) and mediating processes. The

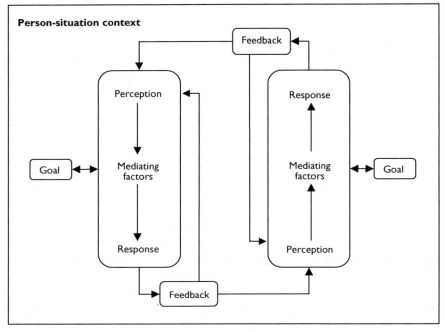

Figure 3.2 Hargie's model of interpersonal communication

latter are processes that mediate between the goal being pursued, our perceptions of events and what we decide to do about them. They also play a
part in the formation of goals, influence how people and events are perceived, and reflect the capacity of the individual to assimilate, deal with and
respond to the particular circumstances of social encounters. Mediating
processes include various cognitive processes (such as semantic encoding,
organization, storage and retrieval of information, inferential processes and
response generation), as well as affective processes, and our perception of
others and of self.

Models of health behaviour

Given that this book is about health communication, we next look at two of
the main social cognition models of health behaviour. Social cognition
models in general have been developed in an attempt to explain, predict and
influence health behaviours and outcomes. They are based on the assumption that people make behaviour decisions on the basis of their beliefs. The
two models to be considered here further assume that choices between
different courses of action are determined by two types of cognition:

subjective probabilities that a given action will lead to a set of expected outcomes, and evaluation of the outcomes. They are rational reasoning models, in that people are believed to consider consciously the different consequences of the various options before deciding whether or not to engage in particular health behaviours.

The Health Belief Model

The Health Belief model was originally proposed by Rosenstock (1966) and was further developed by Becker and Rosenstock (1984) in the 1970s and 1980s. This model was the first analysis of decisions concerning health behaviours that emphasized that such decisions are a function of people's subjective perceptions about a potential health threat and a relevant behaviour. According to the model, perceived threat motivates people to take action, but beliefs about potential behaviours determine the specific plan of attack. Threat is operationalized in terms of both perceptions of the severity of a particular health problem and perceptions of the person's susceptibility to that health problem. This means that effective health communications need to emphasize both of these factors in order to influence health beliefs. Relevant beliefs concern the perceived benefits of taking appropriate action as well as any perceived barriers to taking that action. The final element in the model (as shown in Figure 3.3) specifies that behaviour is driven by internal (e.g. bodily symptoms) or external (e.g. a mass media campaign) cues to action.

The Health Belief Model has been applied to a variety of health behaviours, including smoking, dieting and exercise (see Sheeran and Abraham, 1996, for a review). A number of studies have provided support

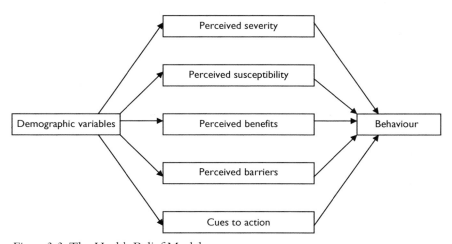

Figure 3.3 The Health Belief Model

for the model. Research has shown, for example, that health behaviours such as eating a healthy diet and taking regular exercise are related to individual beliefs that the health concern is severe, that they are susceptible to it and that the benefits of adopting the health behaviour will outweigh any costs (e.g. Harrison et al., 1992). However, other studies have reported conflicting findings (e.g. Jenz and Becker, 1984). The primary criticism of the model is that the effects of the model's constructs, in terms of accurately predicting health behaviours, tend to be fairly small (e.g. Rutter and Quine, 2002), and that the model takes a rather static approach to health beliefs and does not sufficiently consider the temporal dynamic aspects (Schwarzer, 1992). Overall, the evidence suggests that although the beliefs specified by the model are prerequisites for preventative health behaviours, other cognitions are likely to be involved in prompting such behaviours. In addition, social and economic variables and emotional factors, such as fear (leading to avoidance), may play a part.

The Theory of Planned Behaviour

Although health beliefs go some way towards helping us to understand when people will change their health behaviours, it is also now recognized that a complete model of health behaviour needs to pay more attention to the role of behavioural intentions and actions. The Theory of Planned Behaviour (Azjen, 1985, 1988) attempts to link health beliefs directly to behaviour. It proposes that intentions should be conceptualized as plans of action in pursuit of behavioural goals. Intentions result from three factors or beliefs, these being, the attitude towards the behaviour, subjective norms (including social norms and pressures) and perceived behavioural control or self-efficacy. According to the model, these three factors predict behavioural intentions, which are then linked to behaviour. However, it also acknowledges that perceived behavioural control can have a direct effect on behaviour itself (as shown in Figure 3.4). This means that in order to influence health behaviours, health communications need to address these three factors.

In general, empirical studies have shown that the Theory of Planned Behaviour can predict a broad array of health behaviours, including exercise, vitamin taking, sunscreen use and contraceptive use. Armitage and Conner (2000) reviewed 185 studies that had been carried out, and found that the theory accounted for around 40 per cent of the variance in behavioural intentions and 27 per cent of the variance in actual behaviours. Although the Theory of Planned Behaviour has received less criticism than the Health Belief model, some researchers have pointed out that a significant weakness of the model is that, like the Health Belief model, it does not include a temporal element (e.g. Rutter and Quine, 2002). Other critics have argued that the model is too subjective, it neglects important social variables, and it does not specify the relationship between the different health beliefs (e.g. Schwartzer, 1992).

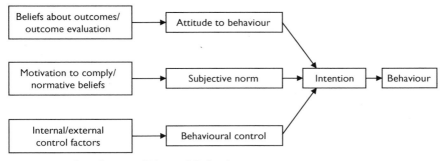

Figure 3.4 The Theory of Planned Behaviour

Northouse and Northouse's model of health comm. unciation

So far we have looked at general theories and models of communication and social cognition models of health behaviour. The next model we will look at, Northouse and Northouse's (1998) model of health communication, specifically considers communication in the context of health. According to Northouse and Northouse, health communication refers to transactions between participants in healthcare and about health-related issues. The model emphasizes the way in which a series of factors (most notably, relationships, transactions and contexts) can impact on the interactions in healthcare settings.

As can be seen in Figure 3.5, the model illustrates the four major types of relationship that exist in healthcare settings: professional–professional, professional–client, professional–client's significant others and client–significant others. Both health professionals and clients bring unique characteristics, beliefs, values and perceptions to the healthcare setting, which affect how they interact. The client's significant others (such as family, friends, work colleagues) are included in the model because they have been found to play a significant role in supporting clients in relation to their health.

The second major element in Northouse and Northouse's model is transactions; that is, the health-related interactions that occur between participants. Health transactions include both verbal and non-verbal communications, as well as the content and relationship dimensions of messages. According to Northouse and Northouse, the relationship dimension of health transactions is established within the various relationships represented by the model, and this dimension influences how the content of the messages should be interpreted. The central spiral depicted in Figure 3.5 illustrates the ongoing transactional and interactive nature of health communication, whereby the different participants influence each other's communications as an interaction progresses.

A third major element in the model is healthcare contexts; that is, the

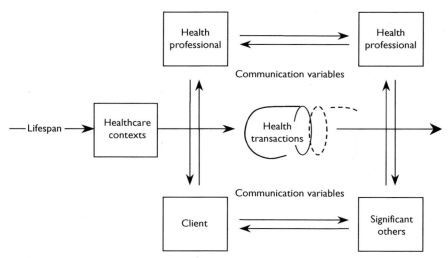

Figure 3.5 Northouse and Northouse's model of health communication

settings in which health communication occurs. As noted in Chapter 2, different contexts have been shown to have a significant influence on the form and effectiveness of communications between the different participants. Contexts can refer to particular settings (such as waiting rooms and hospital wards), or to the number of participants within the particular setting.

Transactional Analysis

As we just saw, transactions are a key element in the Northouse and Northouse model. One way of analysing such transactions is to use Transactional Analysis (e.g. Berne, 1958). Thus, rather than being a formal model as such, Transactional Analysis is a method through which most forms of interpersonal communication can be systematically analysed. It can also be used as a tool for therapeutic intervention. According to this approach, the basic unit of intercourse is called a transaction. Thus, in simple communicative situations, one person initiates an interaction with a transaction stimulus. In turn, a second person's response is known as the transaction response. Fundamental to the approach are three basic ego states (the Child, Parent and Adult states). It is assumed that we all have a different mixture of the three states, and that their presence affects communication in a given situation, depending on which state or combination of states predominates at that time. The Child ego state is one in which emotions or reactions are on the surface, and therefore the state tends to take over at times of high emotion. In contrast, the Parent ego state is one in which we behave like a figure with status who directs the life of others and who establishes standards and values. Finally, the Adult ego state is one which is characterized by detachment and logic; the adult is thus an information handler and decision maker.

Transactional Analysis specifies five different types of transaction that involve an exchange between various combinations of the ego states in our interactions:

1 Complementary transactions: this is where the Adult ego states of both people interact with one another. Although the styles match to some extent, the situation can sometimes lead to breakdown in communications.
2 Crossed transactions: this is where a message sent from one ego state gets an unexpected response, which is often negative and critical.
3 Angular transactions: this is where a speaker talks as if to one ego state but is covertly addressing another state.
4 Ulterior transactions: these involve more than two ego states at the same point in time.
5 Duplex transactions: these involve two messages being transmitted at the same time, where the first is overt and carries a different meaning from the second (more covert) message.

Another key notion is that of hungers (i.e. communication needs) that underlie all transactions and the development of ego states. According to the approach, social interaction is organized by people over periods of time in various ways. Thus, time periods can be short term (described as rituals, games, etc.) or long term (described as scripts). Games are blocks of inter-action in which one person tries to manipulate another person or persons, in order to gain some psychological advantage. Although they have pay-offs for individuals, they can be negative and destructive to relationships, as they are about dominance and submission in relationships. Scripts also have pay-offs for the user but are seen as the blueprint of a person's life map; that is, the structure of a person's life from birth to and through adulthood. They can be thought of as model stories that get carried in the head and that influence all interactions. It has been suggested that effective communication skills involve refusing to play games and recognizing life scripts.

Models of persuasion

The goal of communication can take many different forms, including the elimination of an existing belief, changing the strength of a particular belief, creation of a new belief, changing an intention to carry out an action and changing actual behaviour. Many of those can be classed as aspects of persuasion. In general, persuasion refers to any change in attitudes that results from exposure to communication. Given that much of health communication involves trying to persuade people to adopt particular health behaviours, the final section of this chapter will review two influential models of persuasion: the Elaboration Likelihood Model and the Heuristic Systematic Model. Both can be characterized as being dual-process models as they both involve the use of two different processing modes or routes.

The Elaboration Likelihood Model

The Elaboration Likelihood Model (ELM) was developed by Petty and Cacioppo (1986). According to this model, persuasion occurs via one of two different processes, with the selected one depending on the amount of elaboration or scrutiny required. Petty and Cacioppo defined elaboration as 'the extent to which a person thinks about the issue relevant arguments contained in a message' (1986, p. 128). Elaboration can be thought of as falling along a continuum. At one end there is an enormous amount of cognitive activity, as people think about and elaborate on the message arguments. At the other end, in contrast, there is very little thinking about these arguments, and decisions are made on other grounds. The model states that a message can change attitudes (or produce resistance to change) by getting a person to think hard about the points being made (using central processing) or by inducing them to focus on simple but compelling cues that are usually not central to the message content (using the peripheral route). Thus central processing is characterized by cognitive elaboration and deliberation. In contrast, peripheral processing is more superficial and characterized by an association of the advocated position with other factors, such as the attractiveness or credibility of the message source. This latter route is also associated with the use of simple heuristics or decision rules, such as 'never trust a politician', or 'statistics never lie'.

In terms of health communication, many (although not all) one-to-one interactions between doctors and patients (particularly where serious health issues are being discussed) will involve patients using the central route, in that the participants will tend to think carefully about what the doctor is saying. At the other extreme, however, one can see that health-related advertising and some public health campaigns often rely on people being swayed by more superficial aspects of the communication, such as the attractiveness of the person giving the message, and other associated features.

Clearly, the extent to which one or other route is used will depend on particular factors. The model stipulates that two factors that have a large effect are the individual's motivation level and their ability to process the message. Motivation is primarily affected by the extent to which a person has involvement with the particular issue (for example, when the message relates to a newly diagnosed medical condition). Thus, it is argued that, under high involvement, people will engage in more issue-relevant thinking (that is, use the central route). Similarly, use of the central route is more likely to occur when people feel more able to process the information effectively. A final aspect of the model is that attitudes formed via the central route are thought to show longer persistence over time and more resistance to counter-arguments than those formed via the peripheral route.

Although most characterizations of the Elaboration Likelihood Model refer to the use of one or other processing route, in practice it is likely that many situations will involve people using both routes. There is no reason, for example, why a careful well-constructed set of arguments cannot be delivered by a particularly attractive message source. A good deal of research has been carried out to test the model. In general, such research has provided support for the model when a limited number of variables are examined per study (for example, message source and argument quality). However, the model's effectiveness has been more difficult to judge when complexity has been increased (Petty and Cacioppo, 1986).

The Heuristic Systematic Model

The Heuristic Systematic Model (HSM) was first put forward by Chaiken and colleagues (e.g. Bohner et al., 1995; Chaiken, 1980, 1987). As mentioned earlier, it is similar to the ELM as both models involve the use of two different ways of processing messages. Chaiken and colleagues refer to these as systematic and heuristic processing. Systematic processing involves the use of cognitive resources and is said to occur when people make a judgement by carefully examining, comparing and relating arguments. In this mode, people may exert considerable effort in a search for information and a scrutiny of arguments. Again it is argued that people need to be motivated in order to do this. However, if unmotivated, they will use a less demanding mode of processing. Thus, with heuristic processing, people do not engage in careful reasoning but instead use simple cognitive heuristics (mental short-cuts or rules of thumb). For example, they may believe that longer arguments are stronger or more credible, or be influenced by so-called expert opinion or social consensus or rely on old adages such as 'statistics never lie'. Clearly, this route requires less effort and fewer cognitive resources. As with the preceding model, it is assumed that judgements reached via heuristic processing tend to be less stable and less tied to subsequent behaviour than judgements reached via systematic processing.

The balance of heuristic and systematic processing occurs through the operation of a sufficiency principle, whereby a person engages in enough systematic processing to ensure that his or her actual level of confidence in the position being advocated in the message is higher than his or her desired level of confidence. As with the ELM, the two types of processing are regarded as endpoints on a continuum. However, the relationship between them is not symmetrical. When people are using systematic processing, they may also use heuristics elements. However, when processing heuristically, they will not be engaging in much systematic processing. There are other differences between the ELM and HSM, in that the ELM's peripheral route encompasses more than does HSM's heuristic processing. However, HSM involves a broader interpretation of what motivates people, in that motivation may stem from a desire for confirmatory evidence and accuracy, but it may also stem from a desire to safeguard particular self-concepts or a need to project a particular self-image. In addition, it is believed that not only our cognitions but also our emotions affect which processing mode we use. Mackie and Worth (1989), for example, found that merely being in a good mood may make us less likely to use systematic processing. Similarly, Schmidt and Brewer (2000) found that mood affected the way in which jurors processed information in a mock jury setting. Overall, while there are differences between the HSM and the ELM, research studies have provided support for both, particularly for the use of heuristics and the importance of prior knowledge (e.g. Biek et al., 1996; Petty et al., 1997).

Summary

This chapter has reviewed a number of theories and models that have been put forward to explain the way we communicate and what influences our communications and health behaviours. These include different approaches to communication, models of health behaviour and health communication, Transactional Analysis, and models of persuasion. The next chapter moves from theories to empirical evidence and looks in more detail at the interactions that occur between the different 'players' in the healthcare process (such as, doctors, nurses, patients, family members, etc.). It reviews much of the research on the different types of communication that take place in both one-to-one and small-group settings.

Communication between patients and health professionals

As we saw in Chapter 1, good communication is central to effective health-care. Communication and information provision play key roles in determining whether people engage in recommended health behaviours and whether the behaviours have a positive outcome. Health communicators may want to achieve any of a number of goals, including providing information, instruction or reassurance, influencing opinions and attitudes, and changing behaviour. Edwards and Hugman (1997, p. 223) identified six core issues that need to be taken into account when planning any health communication:

1 The purpose of the message
2 The state of mind of the intended recipient(s), including their cognitive abilities and emotional state
3 The general context or climate in which the message will be received
4 The medium of communication to be used
5 Feedback mechanisms to assess the effects of the message
6 Monitoring and evaluation.

In most situations, healthcare professionals will need to take account of many, if not all, of these factors when planning their communications with patients and others.

Communication can, and does, take place between any of a number of different players in the healthcare process. This chapter is concerned with one-to-one and small-group interactions in healthcare. Chapter 7 looks at communication with the wider public. There are numerous different types of relationship in the healthcare process. In each case, communication is affected by the role each person plays and their expectations of others (and themselves). The quality of the relationship that exists, or develops, during healthcare interactions has an important influence on the smoothness and effectiveness on the communication.

Communication in relationship building

Successful medical encounters will usually depend on developing and maintaining effective relationships, which in turn depend on effective communication between the different participants. According to Burton and Dimbleby (1995), all relationships are conceived, affirmed, conducted and even broken by the use of communication. Communication is used to establish information about others to reduce uncertainty. Relationships are developed through degrees of self-disclosure, in which participants gradually reveal information, attitudes and feelings through communication. The quality of the relationship depends on the positive use of social and perceptual skills. Empathy and trust are important for building positive relationships, whereas game playing can have detrimental effects. Empathy involves trying to feel with the other person in order to understand their point of view. Trust involves accepting others without judging them, and believing that they are basically sincere, competent and accepting. As a result of such trust, individuals should be able to rely on the communicative behaviours of others. Without trust, even the most effective of communications is unlikely to bring about the desired effects. In healthcare settings, trust is particularly important, as many patients and family members often feel helpless and vulnerable. Trust is enhanced when health providers use supportive communicative behaviours, whereas it can be hindered by the use of defensive behaviours. As Hargie and Dickson (2004) noted, health professionals should not assume that patients will automatically trust them as a result of their status. It is important to foster trust and credibility, by attending to patients' needs and communicative behaviours appropriately, and then to maintain them. It has frequently been commented that it can take a long time to build trust, but trust can be lost in a brief moment.

Communication in healthcare encounters

As noted by Street (2003), medical consultations, like other types of social interactions, are dynamic, creative and, usually, socially constructed events. The primary activity is typically 'talk', as the different partners exchange information, make decisions and establish or maintain a relationship. The nature and quality of the interaction will depend on how participants select, adapt and co-ordinate their responses in order to achieve desired goals.

Edelmann (2000) suggested that most clinical encounters can be thought of as an interaction between two distinct 'cultures' – the medical culture and the culture of the patient. The two groups often think differently about health and illness, and have different perceptions, attitudes, knowledge and agendas. The patient's agenda will reflect their own unique experience of illness and their ideas and expectations about consultation and treatment, whereas the healthcare provider's will reflect his or her (usually Western) medical or other health-related training, as well as personal background factors. According to Roter and Hall (1989), most healthcare encounters have two basic goals: those that involve instrumental tasks such as information giving and question asking, and those that involve socio-emotional tasks such as partnership building. They suggested that the two types of task are related to different outcomes, in that adherence and recall tend to be indicators or outcomes of instrumental task-related features, whereas patient satisfaction is more associated with socio-emotional aspects of interactions.

Different participants in healthcare encounters will have different communicative styles. Research has shown that individual healthcare providers vary in terms of how often they provide information, use partnership building and display reassurance. Key factors that influence this include the provider's age, sex, level of education, personality and values. Thus, for example, women doctors have been found to spend longer with patients, and to spend more time addressing their social and emotional needs (e.g. Roter and Hall, 2004). Despite these general differences, it has also been noted that healthcare providers tend to adapt their style of interaction in consistent ways according to the nature of the patient. Thus, for example, healthcare providers often use a more serious manner, focus more on physical and technical aspects, and assume more control with patients who are more seriously ill. Similarly, as we will see in the next chapter, they may well adapt their style of interaction according to the patient's age.

Individual patients will also differ in their style of interaction depending on such things as their age, sex, ethnic background, level of education, and personality. Not surprisingly, these differences affect the nature and quality of interactions. Several studies have reported, for example, that patients who frequently ask questions and offer opinions generally receive more information and elicit more support and reassurance from healthcare providers than those who participate less. We look at the effects of some of these patient factors more in Chapter 5.

Northouse and Northouse (1998) noted that, in addition to specific personal and professional characteristics, relationships between healthcare providers and patients are affected by four factors that can act as potential barriers to effective communication and relationship building. These are: uncertainty over the particular 'role' that patients are expected to play; uncertainty over who is responsible for managing particular aspects of the patient's illness and care; asymmetrical 'power' relationships (where the health professional usually has more power); and the fact that healthcare providers tend to use medical jargon that is unfamiliar to patients. In addition, Davis and Fallowfield (1994) suggested that the majority of communication problems that occur in healthcare interactions involve health professionals making some very basic mistakes. This includes not introducing themselves, not asking for clarification from patients, not allowing or encouraging patients to ask questions, not asking about patients' feelings and not providing information in a form that patients can use.

As with other professions, medicine tends to have its own specialist language, and healthcare professionals and patients are likely to differ in the way they express themselves. Although healthcare providers can potentially switch from medical to everyday language, they tend to over-rely on medical jargon, which patients often have difficulty understanding. Hadlow and Pitts (1991), for example, found that patients only understood 36 per cent of terms that were commonly used by health professionals. The use of technical language is particularly problematic as studies have shown that the use of more technical messages is associated with less cognitive satisfaction, comprehension and recall (e.g. Jackson, 1992). At the other extreme, some healthcare professionals resort to using patronizing language, almost 'baby talk', when interacting with patients, particularly older adults, adolescents and some ethnic groups (see Chapter 5). As with over-reliance on medical jargon and technical language, talking down to patients also results in frustration, lack of satisfaction, and poorer health outcomes.

Doctor–patient communication

According to Ong et al. (1995), the doctor–patient relationship is one of the most complex interpersonal relationships. It involves the interaction between people in non-equal positions, is often non-voluntary, concerns issues of vital importance, is emotionally laden and requires close co-operation. In evaluating patterns of control and communication in doctor–patient relationships, Roter and Hall (1992) described four basic forms: default, paternalistic, consumerist and mutualistic. Default relationships are characterized by a lack of control on either side, and are clearly far from ideal. Paternalism is characterized by dominant doctors and passive patients, whereas consumerism is associated with the reverse, with it focusing on patients' rights and doctors' obligations. Finally, mutuality is characterized by a sharing of decision making and is often advocated as the best type of relationship. It may not suit all types of patient, however, and is often difficult to achieve in practice.

As Fallowfield et al. (2002) emphasized, effective communication between doctors and patients can have many beneficial effects. Thus, it is an important determinant of the accuracy and completeness of data collection about symptoms and side effects, dictates the problems elicited, affects adherence to treatment recommendations, influences emotional and physical well-being, and contributes to satisfaction of both patients and clinicians.

Edelmann (2000) identified four main factors that are likely to influence the nature and effectiveness of doctor–patient interactions:

1 The characteristics of the doctor (particularly his or her sex, and level of experience)

2 The characteristics of the patient (including, sex, social class, age, education and desire for information)
3 Differences between the two parties in terms of social class and education, attitudes, beliefs and expectations
4 Situational factors (such as patient load, level of acquaintance and nature of the presenting problem).

Many patients experience some degree of apprehension, and even anxiety, when visiting a doctor, and the extent of this will also influence their interactions. Admission to hospital can be a particularly disturbing experience. In such cases, patients often finds themselves in an unfamiliar environment, separated from family and friends, with a loss of personal space, privacy and independence, and often feeling uncertain about their health problem and its treatment. These factors often lead to them feeling very vulnerable, and are likely to affect the way they interact with health professionals.

Interestingly, doctors and patients have very different perspectives on the factors that they see as being most important in doctor–patient communication. Paling (2004) described a simple research project that asked doctors and patients, what in their view makes a good doctor. The doctors stated that 'diagnostic ability' was the most important quality of a good doctor, whereas the patients said that 'listening' was the most important aspect. This latter aspect was rated as being least important by the doctors. The findings are in line with an earlier study by Delamothe (1998), which found that the top three categories for what most influences a patient's choice of good doctor were 'how well the doctor communicates with patients and shows a caring attitude', 'explaining medical or technical procedures in an easy-to-understand way' and 'listening and taking the time to ask questions'. In contrast, the aspects most highly rated by doctors were 'number of years of practice' and 'whether the doctor had attended a well known medical school'.

A recent empirical study by Corke et al. (2005) showed that doctors' bias towards spending more time covering technical medical issues is reflected in practice. They carried out an observational study of doctor–patient interviews based on a standardized clinical scenario, involving high-risk surgery and a hypothetical patient with serious co-morbidities (played by an actor). The findings showed that the medical situation was well described by nearly all the doctors, but that the patient's functional status, values and fears were only poorly or minimally addressed. This difference in emphasis is not surprising given that the majority of doctors (particularly in the Western world) have been trained to adopt a very doctor- or disease-centred orientation to consultations, and this approach tends to continue throughout medical careers (Fallowfield, 2002).

Clearly, doctors have to communicate with patients to achieve a number of different goals. In line with this, Ong et al. (1995) suggested that there are three basic different purposes of communication between doctors and patients: creating a good interpersonal relationship, exchange of information and medical decision making. We will consider each in turn.

Creating a good interpersonal relationship

As noted earlier, establishing and maintaining a good relationship is a prerequisite for optimal medical care. A number of studies have shown that a successful doctor–patient relationship and communication can have an important positive effect on factors such as patient satisfaction, knowledge and understanding, adherence to treatment and measurable health outcomes. After reviewing the literature to date, Squirer (1990) concluded that there is strong evidence that the affective quality of the doctor–patient relationship is a key determinant of both patient satisfaction and adherence to treatment. In particular, warmth, caring, positive regard, lack of tension and non-verbal expressiveness appeared to be the most important elements in establishing and maintaining an effective working relationship. Studies have demonstrated that practitioners' affective behaviours, such as showing concern and empathy, play an important role in encouraging patients to disclose their emotions and discuss genuine concerns (e.g. Culos-Reed et al., 2000; Roter, 2000). Williams et al. (1998) reported that increased patient satisfaction was related to the doctor's friendliness, courteous behaviour, social conversation, encouraging and empathic behaviours, and partnership building, as well as to higher patient centredness and expression of empathy during consultations. Similarly, Roter et al. (1998) found that adherence to treatment was greater among patients whose doctors expressed encouragement, resassurance and support. In terms of actual health outcomes, Stewart (1995) carried out a meta-review of 21 studies in the literature and showed that quality of doctor–patient communication was found to have a significant influence on patient health outcomes, such as emotional health, symptom resolution, function, physiological measures (for example, decreased blood pressure and blood sugar) and pain control. More recently, Dulmen and Bensing (2001) reported that an empathic interaction was more likely to lead to a reduction in anxiety, pain and blood pressure (Bensing and Verhaak, 2004).

Unfortunately, there is also evidence that that not all doctor–patient relationships are as positive as many patients would like. Roberts et al. (2001), for instance, noted that the manner of communication between doctors and patients is still a major cause of patient dissatisfaction. Most complaints about doctors by patients concern poor communication and failure to listen, rather than their actual competence or the more technical aspects of consultations.

Exchange of information

The second purpose of doctor–patient communication outlined by Ong et al. (1975) is exchange of information. From the medical point of view, doctors need to elicit information from patients in order to establish the right diagnosis and treatment plan. From the other perspective, patients need to know and understand and to feel known and understood. In order to fulfil both needs, the two parties need to alternate between information giving and seeking. As noted by Noble (1998), the manner in which doctors elicit information from their patients at the start of consultations can, and does, determine the eventual outcome. A number of studies have shown that doctors tend to 'over control' consultations, particularly by frequently interrupting patients. Beckman and Frankel (1984), for example, reported that patients were interrupted on average only 18 seconds after starting their description of the problem, and that only 23 per cent of them actually completed their intended statements (see also Epstein et al., 1993). Similarly, Roter and Hall (1989) reported that the doctors in their study elicited less than 50 per cent of the medical information available from patients. Not surprisingly, patients' inputs to medical consultations are influenced by the doctor's style of interaction. Street (2003), for instance, observed that patients tend to ask more questions, express opinions more freely, provide more psychosocial information and discuss concerns more openly when doctors use partnership building and other types of patient-centred responses.

As far as information giving is concerned, a number of studies have found that doctors commonly underestimate the amount of information about their illnesses and treatments that patients want. According to Donovan and Blake (1992), for instance, most rheumatoid arthritis patients in their study craved more information about their disease and treatments than they were given. In particular, they wanted information about aetiology, symptoms, methods of diagnosis, likely prognosis of disease, nature and effects on symptoms/disease and side effects of drugs, as well as information on treatment options and self-help techniques available. Similarly, Coulter et al. (1998) found that patients wanted much more information about their condition and treatments than they had been given. Most had not been offered choice about their treatments, nor even realized that there were options.

More recently, Elder and Suter (2005) found that 85 per cent of preadmission patients about to undergo cataract surgery requested additional written information about their treatments, particularly about the risks and benefits involved. As indicated, in practice, not all patients receive the amount or type of information they would like. Williams (1993), for instance, found that more than 30 per cent of hospital patients in their study reported receiving no information about their anaesthesia, time in operating theatre, likely pain that will be experienced and the time-course of their return to fitness. Similarly, Kerzman et al. (2005) reported that, although most patients discharged from a large hospital in Israel were aware of the course and purpose of their medicine, very few were aware of potential side effects, necessary lifestyle changes and correct medication schedules. Thus,

LIBRARY, UNIVERSITY OF CHESTER

as Noble (1998) previously noted, many patients lack even the most basic information about their treatments. In one sense this is surprising as research has consistently shown that doctors who provide clear information, especially when coupled with emotional support, are more likely to obtain positive patient outcomes such as reduced psychological stress, enhanced symptom resolution and reduced blood pressure (e.g. Roter, 2000; Roter et al., 2001). As we will see in Chapter 6, effective information provision is also an integral part of obtaining truly informed consent from patients for their treatments and/or participation in clinical research trials.

Medical decision making

Finally, the third purpose of communication identified by Ong et al. (1995) is medical decision making. Over the past 20 years or so, there has been a marked shift from what has been termed a 'paternalistic' model of medicine, whereby doctors made all the decisions, to a more patient-centred model, in which the decision making is shared between doctors and patients. Patient-centred medicine stresses the importance of understanding patients' experiences of their illnesses, as well as relevant social and psychological factors. It involves the doctor employing active listening skills (see Chapter 8), attempting to understand the patient's point of view and working with patients to find common ground regarding treatment management. Coulter (1999) suggested that the key to successful doctor–patient relationships and decision making is recognizing that patients are experts too. Doctors may well be informed about causes of disease, prognosis, treatment options and preventative strategies, but only the patient knows about his or her illness, social circumstances, habits, attitudes to risks, values and preferences. In line with this, shared decision making therefore involves a two-way exchange of information, whereby both the doctor and the patient discuss treatment preferences and agree on which option(s) to try. Doctors need to establish an atmosphere in which patients feel that their views are valued and needed. Charles et al. (1997) identified four main characteristics of shared decision making; these being, involvement of both the patient and doctor, a sharing of information by both parties, both parties taking steps to build consensus about the preferred treatment and reaching an agreement about which treatment to implement.

Research has shown that increased patient involvement and shared decision making does produce beneficial results. Crawford et al. (2002) reviewed the relevant literature on the effects of involving patients in healthcare planning and decision making in a range of settings and found that higher levels of involvement resulted in better quality of care, increased satisfaction (for both patients and medical stafff), and improved self-esteem for patients. However, it has been noted that not all patients want to participate in decision making about their healthcare. Such reluctance tends to be more prevalent in older patients and those who are more seriously ill. In such cases, doctors may need to use a more directive approach, but they should still ensure that they provide all the relevant information that is wanted, or needed, by the patient.

Communication between patients and other healthcare professionals

Although there are many similarities between the healthcare interactions of doctors and patients and other healthcare providers and patients, some differences have been observed. Thus, for example, where the health professional is perceived by the patient to be of a 'less high status', such as is often the case with nurses, it has been noted that patients may be more open and more likely to ask questions and volunteer more information about their illness, feelings and concerns.

Heaven (1997) observed that doctors' conversations with patients and relatives may differ from those of their professional colleagues for a number of reasons. A key reason is that each professional has a different area of interest and different skills and expertise. Thus, doctors who have a high level of training in anatomy and physiology frequently focus communications on biomedical symptoms and forming a diagnosis and appropriate treatment plan. A nurse, in contrast, may be more likely to consider the impact of the illness on the patient and his or her family. The focus is likely to be more on care and developing a care plan.

Another reason for different healthcare professionals having different conversations with patients and family members is that, as noted earlier, patients and relatives often choose to interact differently with different types of professional. Studies, for example, have shown that patients disclose different types and amounts of information to different medical carers (e.g. Cole-Kelly, 1992). Given these different experiences, it is essential that healthcare professionals meet regularly to discuss and exchange information about the patients they are treating in order to obtain the fullest picture.

In recent years, many healthcare professionals have found themselves having to cope with changing, usually more expanded, roles. For example, both nurses and pharmacists are now able to prescribe to patients a large number of medicines that were previously only prescribed by doctors. Studies have shown that most health professionals and patients are now comfortable with these expanded roles (e.g. Berry et al., 2006; Latter and Courtenay, 2004; Luker et al., 1998). Berry et al. (2006), for example, recently carried out an empirical study, with a sample of the general population, and found that the majority were happy to be prescribed medicines by nurses and saw a number of advantages for themselves (such as ease of access, greater continuity of care and better information provision) as well as for health professionals (for example, increased nurse status and job satisfaction, and allowing doctors more time for complicated or demanding cases). These extended roles, as they are known, can however place pressure on communications. Health professionals who take on these roles may have to provide more technical information than they are used to, and may on occasion find themselves in situations where they might want to express views that are in conflict with those of the doctors involved in the case.

Communication between healthcare providers and patients' families

Patients rarely exist and experience ill health in a vacuum. It has become increasingly apparent in recent years that patients' families, friends and other carers play an important role in relation to supporting patients and increasing the chance that positive health outcomes will be obtained. Bloom (1996), for example, noted that patients' 'significant others' were a key factor in mediating various life stresses and serious illnesses. Similarly, Mannes et al. (1993) observed that significant individuals, such as family members, affect patients' health behaviours, ability to cope with illness and treatment adherence.

Each family member will cope with, and adjust to, a relative's illness in a different way depending on their role and the relationships that exist within the family. Having to communicate with different family members, with different levels of knowledge and different emotional states, can clearly be challenging for healthcare professionals. Enquiries from family members can also cause difficulties because relatives often approach, and seek information from, several different members of healthcare teams, particularly junior and more 'vulnerable' members, in an attempt to try to get at the truth. Family members may or may not then pass this information on to the patient, depending on whether they feel it would be in their and the patient's best interests. Despite these potential difficulties, Northouse and Northouse (1998) pointed out that, if more attention is given to the needs of family members and friends, these significant others will be able to join forces with staff to support the patient to achieve healthcare goals. They stressed that if family and friends are to maintain their supportive role in healthcare, they need to have effective communications from, and with, health professionals. However, they noted that this can be impeded by two key factors: the fact that they often have limited contact with health professionals and that their access to information can be limited. Problems can be caused, or exacerbated, by both parties. Family members have been noted to be reluctant to ask for help as they do not want to take up any of the professional's time. Ryan (1992) showed that family members ranked the patient's needs as being higher than their own and did not want to divert doctors and other health professionals from attending to these. However, studies have also shown that family members and other caregivers sometimes receive little acknowledgement from health professionals, and are often excluded from discussions and decision making about the patient's welfare even when they play a key role in caring for the patient (e.g. Stetz et al., 1996).

As far as access to information is concerned, Northouse and Northouse (1998) pointed out that problems can be of two sorts: privileged communication and filtered communication. The former occurs because, in some instances, family members are provided with information by healthcare providers that has not been given to patients. This is less common now than was once the case (and is less common in our culture than in some others), but family members are sometimes still told certain key information before it is given to patients. Filtered information refers to information that family and friends receive from the patient or other non-professional sources. Given that we know that patients do not understand, or forget, much of what they are told in medical consultations, there are clearly problems when family and other caregivers have to rely on this source of information in order to determine how best to support the patient.

Communication between different healthcare professionals

Communication with patients and their families will differ in many respects from communications between different healthcare professionals. Different types of professional will have different skills and expertise, and will often have different experience of, and insight into, a particular patient's medical problems. It has been noted in the literature that healthcare providers need to collaborate and co-operate with each other in order to benefit patient care. However, it has also been observed that effective teamwork and collegiality are not always evident. Northouse and Northouse (1998) identified three different problem areas: role stress, a lack of inter-professional understanding and autonomy struggles. Role stress can occur when there is a conflict between the roles professionals are expected to take and their own personal values and beliefs, when professionals have to take on duties and tasks that they perceive are not directly related to their primary role, and when there is role overload, for example when numbers of referrals are too large or too unpredictable.

Lack of inter-professional understanding may at first seem surprising. However, traditional medical education and other healthcare training have been very 'profession based', with different professional groups being educated in isolation from other groups, and with little opportunity to learn about other providers' skills, roles and responsibilities. This is now starting to change, with the introduction of inter-professional education, but it is still early days. In addition to background educational factors, in many medical settings there is only relatively limited contact between different healthcare professionals on a day-to-day basis. Katzman and Roberts (1988), for example, studied doctor–nurse communication in a hospital setting and found that there was relatively little routine interaction between the two parties. This does vary from one healthcare setting to another, however. Thus, there may be more inter-professional interaction in community practice settings, for example, than on surgical wards.

The final problem area identified by Northouse and Northouse (1998) – autonomy struggles – refers to the actual or perceived freedom to be self-directing. In general, doctors are perceived to have much more autonomy than many other health professionals, such as nurses and social workers. It has been noted that where differences do exist, the dominant profession often tends to underestimate the professionalism or competence of other healthcare providers, which can lead to interpersonal tension and frustration. Again, such issues tend to be more likely to arise in the traditionally 'hierarchical' areas of medicine, such as surgery, and less likely to occur in areas such as palliative care and in community settings. It is possible that as nurses and other healthcare professionals take on new and expanded roles (such as independent medicine prescribing) autonomy differentials will decrease to some extent.

Good inter-professional working is worth striving for, however, as studies have shown that where working relationships are based on mutual respect and autonomy, this can produce a number of benefits for professionals and patients. These include enhanced patient care (Bredin et al., 1999), a broader range of services being offered (Glajchen et al., 1995), greater job satisfaction (Jenkins, Fallowfield and Poole, 2001) and enhanced support to all those involved in the healthcare process (Oberle and Hughes, 2001).

Communication in small groups in healthcare

An increasing amount of communication in healthcare is now carried out in small groups. As Northouse and Northouse (1998) pointed out, during the past decade or so the healthcare field has seen groups take over functions that were once performed by individuals (or not at all). It is now common practice for working groups to be set up in order to address specific professional practices and issues. In addition, health professionals are increasingly working in multidisciplinary teams which meet to discuss the treatment and support of patients, as well as general healthcare-related issues. From the patient and family perspective, there has been a notable increase in the number of self-help and other support groups that are in existence. These groups can provide effective support for both patients and families and other carers, and have been shown to reduce the load on the healthcare system.

In Chapter 2 we looked at the processes involved in the formation and effective working of small groups, irrespective of the particular context (that is, they would apply equally to healthcare, education and business settings). What is possibly notable about healthcare, however, is the diverse range of types of group likely to be in existence, where the focus, goals and nature of operation may be very different. Small groups in healthcare, as well as in other contexts, tend to differ in terms of whether their primary focus is task oriented or process oriented. The former would include, for example, working groups that have been set up to review current practice in a particular area, such as the operation of a certain clinic or improving the patient pathway in one or more specialisms. Communication within such groups tends to focus very much on goals to be achieved and procedures that need to be adopted. Process–oriented groups, in contrast, tend to focus more on the members themselves and the existing and developing relationships between them. Most self-help and therapeutic groups fall at this end of the continuum. Clearly not all small groups in healthcare fall into one or other category, and many will address task-related and therapeutic goals. Hospital ward meetings, for example, are likely to involve both aspects. The more process oriented a group is, the more essential it is for it to become cohesive. Research has shown that cohesive groups are more likely to be productive, to have consistent membership and to have increased interaction between members. According to Yalom (1995), members of cohesive groups are more likely to feel a sense of belonging and of being valued. Clearly, effective communication between group members, while important in all small groups, is particularly necessary where the focus of the group is more therapeutic and process oriented. Good communication is an essential prerequisite for building and maintaining cohesiveness as, without this, members will not develop trust and interdependence. As we will see in Chapter 8, communication skills training now routinely covers skills that are needed for effective communication in small groups as well as one-to-one settings.

Summary

This chapter has looked at communication between different participants in healthcare encounters. It considered factors that contribute to good relationship building and to effective (and less effective) health communication. The chapter then looked at issues relating to doctor–patient communication, as well as to communication between patients and other healthcare professionals. It also considered communication between healthcare providers and family members, and between different types of provider. Finally, it followed on from Chapter 2 to look at small-group communication in healthcare.

Communicating with particular populations in healthcare

Much of the discussion in the preceding chapters has looked at general features of communication, or at communication between particular types of participant in the healthcare process (such as healthcare professionals or patients). The tendency has been to treat people as being very much the same. Clearly, however, this is not the case, and different communication patterns and issues have been noted to occur in particular sub-groups of the population. The current chapter looks at communicating with some of these 'populations', including older adults, children and parents, people with different ethnic and religious backgrounds, and those who may have low intelligence and other cognitive impairments. Chapter 6 then considers issues relating to communication in particularly difficult circumstances, such as having to convey complex information or bad news, which can occur irrespective of factors such as age, sex and ethnic background.

Communicating with older adults

One group that has been identified in terms of creating challenges for effective communication is older adults. Over the past 20 years or more, particularly in the Western world, we have seen a marked increase in the expected living age, with a resultant increase in the proportion of the population who are over 65 years old. Given that elderly people are, in general, more likely to need healthcare, this is creating a considerable burden on the various healthcare systems that are in place. We know, for example, that people in this age group are more likely to be taking prescribed medication than their younger counterparts (e.g. Cartwright, 1990; McElnay and McCallion, 1998). The *UK National Health Service Framework for Older People* (Department of Health, 2001) indicated that 80 per cent of people over the age of 75 take at least one prescribed medicine, and 36 per cent take four or more. A similar disparity has been noted in other European countries and the USA (e.g. Claesson et al., 1999; Kane et al., 1994; Stewart, 1990). One reason for this heavy reliance on medicine is that older people are more likely to suffer multiple medical problems, many of which are chronic in nature, and require long-term medication.

There is good evidence that communication between healthcare professionals and older adults can be characterized by certain factors. These 'typical communication patterns' tend to be the result of both healthcare professional and patient factors. In general, studies have shown that doctors are often more condescending, abrupt, indifferent and dismissive towards older people (Adelman et al., 1991). They tend to speak louder and in a more patronizing way, often treating older people like young children rather than as fully functioning adults (Jackson and Duffy, 1998). In terms of patient factors, older people tend to ask fewer questions, give less information to healthcare professionals and be less assertive. Studies have also shown that older patients often prefer doctors to be in control, particularly in decision making, and are much less likely to challenge the decisions. As noted by Jackson and Duffy (1998), the greater willingness of older people to 'play by the rules' probably contributes to less effective communication, and ultimately to poorer health outcomes.

According to MacDonald (2004), 'potential barriers to good communication with the elderly are legion' (p. 104). Such barriers may stem from physical and cognitive factors, in addition to the behavioural ones identified earlier. In terms of physical factors, many older people have problems with poor eyesight and hearing loss, as well as physical mobility. Hearing loss can cause particular problems when the communication involves more than two people. Many healthcare professionals are tempted to shout when communicating with those with hearing loss. However, this is not an effective strategy. Rather, it is better to speak slowly, with a low but resonant voice, as most hearing loss is likely to affect perception of higher pitched sounds. Similarly, patients should be seated close to the healthcare provider, and face to face in a good light, so that the patient can read their lips as well as hear their voice. The problems of reduced hearing may be exacerbated because some older people are reluctant to admit to having hearing loss. It is therefore necessary to be sensitive to the possibility of this, even if the patient is not wearing an artificial aid. Written information, that can be taken home by people, is a useful supplement for those with hearing loss, as well as for those with minor cognitive impairments that affect their speed of information processing. However, this should be thought of as a useful supplement to, rather than a replacement for, spoken interaction.

As with hearing loss, the likelihood of cognitive impairment also increases with age. Cognitive impairments can range from being relatively mild (such as in the case of minor forgetfulness) to major (such as with dementia or Alzheimer's disease). Such major impairments are on the increase as the population ages. A BBC news item reported in 2005 (BBC, 2005a) that there were currently 24 million sufferers across the world, and that it was predicted that the rate would double every 20 years. When communicating directly with those who have some degree of cognitive impairment it is necessary to allow time for the patient to process and understand the information or questions, and to respond appropriately. Healthcare professionals should not adopt patronizing 'baby talk' however. Rather they should use familiar terms and simple sentence structures wherever possible. When giving instructions, such as how to use a particular device or take medicines, tasks need to be broken down into smaller discrete steps that can be more easily understood and followed.

Another feature of interactions with elderly patients that can contribute to the difficulties is that older patients are often accompanied to consultations by a third party, such as a spouse or child. In such circumstances, healthcare professionals are often tempted to communicate directly with the third party (particularly if they are notably younger) rather than with the patient themselves. Clearly, this will influence the effectiveness of the interaction, and may diminish the patient's feeling of self-worth.

Communicating with younger children and parents

At the other end of the age span, paediatric care can also present a particular challenge for health communication. Clearly it is not possible to predict or avoid all situations and discussions that may be problematic or stressful for children and parents. However, as noted by Edwards (2004), it is possible to identify good general principles for effective communication that will enhance the quality of the child and family's relationship with, and satisfaction with, the healthcare team. Such principles need to take account of the fact that children vary considerably in terms of the level of their cognitive and emotional maturity. They also have to recognize the, sometimes conflicting, needs of the children and those of their parents and other family members.

Evidence has shown that children do not think about health and illness in the same way as adults. They have different conceptions of their bodies that change as the child goes through different stages of development (Eiser and Twamley, 1999). These different levels of understanding need to be taken into account when communicating with children. As Dorn (1984) noted,

> how effectively one communicates can affect children's reactions to procedures, compliance and therapy, and knowledge about health and illness . . . how one approaches the child, the techniques used, and the language employed determine the degree of success or failure in these interactions.
>
> (p. 325)

There are many barriers to communicating with, and treating, younger children in particular. Young children may be anxious of strangers and scared by unfamiliar medical environments. They may scream and wriggle when undergoing physical examinations, and doctors may worry about hurting them. Parents will get anxious in such situations and may cause additional strain to interactions. Furthermore, it is often difficult to gauge a young child's level of understanding in order to know how best to explain to them what is going on and provide reassurance.

It has been suggested that by understanding how children conceptualize disease and illness we can begin to understand their comprehension of illness (Nussbaum et al., 2003). Bibace and Walsh (1981) proposed that children's conceptualization of illness lies on a continuum of three levels:

1 Pre-logical (2–6 years), where children conceptualize illness as being caused by a force that is external to them, that they do not really understand
2 Concrete-logical (7–10 years), where children believe that sickness occurs via contamination and that it is transmitted by physical contact
3 Formal-logical (11 and older), where children conceptualize illness as a physiological phenomenon in which external factors affect the functioning of internal bodily parts.

Thus, as noted by Lloyd and Bor (1996), it is important to ensure that conversation is pitched at the child's cognitive level. Lloyd and Bor recommended a number of practical suggestions that can be used to improve consultations. These include learning the child's terminology for their concerns and parts of their anatomy and using this when interacting with them, as well as explaining procedures in order to prepare children for strange noises, smells and painful procedures. Other recommendations include talking in a calm reassuring voice, establishing rapport before touching or examining the child, and putting oneself at the same physical level as the child when examining or talking to them. Children should not be admonished for crying, and health professionals should not try to bribe them into behaving in a particular way. Importantly, healthcare providers should not give false reassurance or make promises that cannot be kept.

Trying to communicate directly with the children themselves is important, even if they are relatively young. Studies have shown that while parents are good at giving details about a child's medical problem, they are less good at describing the child's feelings and how they are responding to what is wrong with them (Eiser and Twamley, 1999). The recent *UK National Services Framework for Children* (NSF, 2003) stipulates that children should be encouraged to be active partners in decisions about their healthcare (although it is recognized that the extent to which this is possible will depend on the child's level of maturity and competence). However, despite the acknowledged importance of speaking directly to children and eliciting information from them, studies of consultations between healthcare professionals and young children have shown that this often does not occur.

Wassmer et al. (2004), for example, studied doctor–child–parent communications in an outpatient setting, and found that children only contributed 4 per cent towards interactions, whereas doctors contributed 61 per cent and parents 35 per cent. The doctors' communications were primarily instrumental (asking questions, giving information) rather than being affective or social.

Clearly, it is difficult for healthcare providers to communicate complex information to children, yet most medical information is complex and difficult to communicate even to adults. As we saw in the previous chapter, even adult patients have difficulty understanding common medical terms (Hadlow and Pitts, 1991). It is important to try to find terms that a child will understand, without descending to 'baby talk' unnecessarily. Information needs to be given in manageable amounts and built upon over successive discussions. As noted by Edwards (2004), information needs to be presented in a simple and accessible way, using a range of techniques including demonstrations, play and visual aids, as appropriate to the child's age and level of understanding.

Another source of difficulty in paediatric consultations is that some parents are reluctant to inform their children about their illnesses and to involve them in medical discussions. Although such parents usually believe that they are behaving in the child's best interest, healthcare professionals should try to work with them to explore the consequences of excluding children from interactions, as opposed to including them. Parents often need time to come to terms with their child's condition themselves before feeling able to cope with discussing the problem with the child and addressing his or her concerns. In addition, parents often feel vulnerable and helpless, and some feel guilty and somehow responsible for what is wrong with their child. It should be realized, however, that in practice, children are often more aware of what is going on than parents realize. Thus, it is likely that if they do not get the information they require from their parents and doctors directly, they will seek other sources. This can result in their gaining information, which may not be fully reliable, in an unsupported and ad hoc manner. When children have information withheld, or are misinformed, this is also likely to impair their trust in the healthcare team. However, we know that the quality of the relationship with healthcare professionals has a significant impact on children's confidence and co-operation with future treatments (Edwards, 2004). Such relationships will not develop if the children do not gain trust in the healthcare team.

Other difficulties can arise when there are disagreements between parents and health professionals over the most appropriate treatment for the child. Such situations are particularly likely to occur when the outcome of the treatment is uncertain or when parents want further medical tests, or a second opinion, before agreeing to treatment. Clearly, maintaining good communications in such circumstances is essential. There may also be disagreements between parents, or between parents and children. Health professionals may need to use their communication skills to play an important mediating role in such cases.

Communicating with adolescents

Adolescence is a difficult time and communication with adolescents can be problematic even in normal circumstances. Many teenagers feel a sense of uncertainty, particularly in relation to their identity, and often experience large mood swings. Problems of communication may well increase when teenagers experience illness and have to undergo treatments, as such circumstances usually increase uncertainty levels and place individuals in unfamiliar environments. By definition, the teenage years span from childhood to adulthood, and it is therefore not sensible to think of adolescents as a single category. Younger teenagers may well want parents involved in all interactions with medical staff, whereas older teenagers may not. Whatever the age, teenagers should be addressed directly by healthcare providers, rather than comments being aimed primarily at parents. As MacDonald (2004) pointed out, it is essential to deal with teenagers as equals, addressing them with respect and particularly to avoid patronizing them. Whenever possible, teenagers need to be given the privacy normally accorded to adult patients.

All patients need to be given time to come to terms with a diagnosis and prepare for treatment, and this is especially the case for adolescents. As also noted by MacDonald (2004), it is not unusual for teenagers to need the same information repeated on several occasions before they can really take it in. Young people often use blocking mechanisms when feeling anxious, and this can impair their initial understanding of the information that they are given. They also often hide their true feelings, appearing to be much more confident than they actually are.

One notable feature of adolescents is that they may be less likely to trust their doctors and other healthcare professionals, and automatically believe what they are told. In this context, it has been noted that teenagers are more likely to trust doctors who are honest with them. In contrast, they will be more sceptical about doctors who try to be 'too friendly' or 'familiar'. Clowers (2000), for example, studied US female teenagers' preferences in relation to medical consultations and found that the teenagers particularly disliked physicians who rushed consultations, behaved badly or who were 'too personal'. They preferred doctors who acted professionally but expressed comfort, humour and understanding, and explained procedures clearly. In line with this, MacDonald (2004) suggested that doctors need to be frank and honest when interacting with adolescents, and that they need to be patient and prepared to give the teenagers time. Importantly, they should adopt an informal, but not too personal, style of interaction.

Communicating with patients from different ethnic backgrounds

Owing to worldwide migration, healthcare professionals are increasingly interacting with people from various ethnic and cultural backgrounds. In the USA, for example, it is predicted that, by 2050, Hispanics will constitute 25 per cent of the population, Blacks 14 per cent, Asians 9 per cent, and American Indians 1 per cent (Kar et al., 2001). There is growing recognition that the way people react to illness is rooted in their broader health belief systems, which in turn are culturally determined. Culture can be broadly defined as the learned beliefs, attitudes, values, rules, norms and behaviours that are common to a group of people (Northouse and Northouse, 1998). It encompasses just about everything that a person has seen, heard or felt since their birth. According to Street (2003), ethnicity and culture may affect providers' and patients' communicative behaviour in at least three ways. First, people from different ethnic backgrounds often speak different languages or dialects or, even when technically speaking the same language, there may still be culture-specific usages of it which result in problems of interpretation. Second, as we will see later, preferred styles of communication may vary across different cultural groups, particularly with respect to assertiveness and expressiveness. Finally, people from different ethnic backgrounds often have different explanatory or personal models of health and illness, and these in turn will influence the course and outcome of medical consultations.

Within the western world, the dominant model of health is one that stems from a biomedical perspective. However, different models exist elsewhere in the world, and many migrants to the Western world bring these alternative explanatory models with them. From the Chinese perspective, for example, health is viewed as the result of a balance between and within various systems both internal and external to the person. Disease is perceived as the consequence of disharmony or disequilibrium, and human suffering is traditionally explained as a result of *ming* or destiny. In contrast, within India the majority of the population use ayurvedic medicine, which is based on Hindu philosophy. According to this view of health and illness, the body is defined in terms of the flow of substances through channels, and sickness occurs when a channel is blocked and the flow is diverted into another channel. When all channels are blocked death is likely to occur. Thus the task of ayurvedic medicine is to identify blockages and to get substances moving again. Finally, within Africa a range of traditional medical systems still continue to flourish. These often include a combination of physical and herbal treatments together with various religious belief systems. These belief systems frequently involve spiritual and magical influences, and the orientation towards medicine tends to be communal rather than individualistic.

Many cultures encompass different religious beliefs. Such religious and other culture-specific beliefs often strongly influence how illness and treatment are perceived and will affect healthcare and health communication in different ways. In Islam (the religion of Muslims), for example, illness is regarded as a test of how strongly a person believes in God. Life and death are merely stages in God's overall plan for humanity, and death is often perceived as just a temporary separation from one's loved ones. Muslims argue that treatment should never be discontinued if there is any chance of life continuing, irrespective of the quality of life, as God might decide to revive the patient (particularly if the patient is a strong believer in God). Within many African and Caribbean communities, blood is viewed as the very life of a person and there is a great reluctance to donate blood or bodily organs.

In several Asian communities, many serious illnesses, such as cancer, have a stigma associated with them and sufferers are often isolated from the community by their families. In some other communities, however, particularly those originating from the Middle East, Far East and Mediterranean, there is a strong sense of duty and commitment to family life. When a family member becomes ill it is a matter for the whole family, not just for the individual. This can create difficulties for healthcare and communication because family members may want to stay with the patient at all times.

In terms of differences in communicative style, Kim et al. (1999) observed that people from individualistic cultures (such as Europeans and Anglo-Americans) tend to have independent self-construals that promote more direct, assertive and expressive communication styles. However, people from collectivist cultures (such as some Asian cultures) have interdependent self-construals that lead to communication styles characterized by indirectness, respect for authority and accommodation to others. In cultures that are family centred (for example, Greek, Italian, Hispanic) withholding bad news is defended culturally as protecting the patient.

Our background culture not only influences our verbal language and general communicative style, but also the more subtle non-verbal aspects of language. We noted in Chapter 2 that there are known differences between cultures in terms of aspects of non-verbal behaviour such as the use of gestures, touch and expected personal distance. Healthcare professionals need to be aware of, and sensitive to, these. In addition, there can be differences in relation to the extent to which emotion is expressed (e.g. through facial expressions) in particular situations. The Japanese, for example, are more likely to mask emotional feelings and feeling pain when in the presence of someone in authority, such as a doctor.

Another challenge for effective health communication is the fact that many members of minority groups, particularly those who grew up in developing countries, may have had little opportunity for education. Tufnell et al. (1994), for example, noted that half of the Bangladeshi population in Leeds could not read or write in English, and over a third could not do so in Bengali either. The problems were particularly notable in the older members of the population. This not only hinders interactions but also means that such patients are not likely to benefit from supplementary written information materials.

Studies have shown that the differences in cultural understandings, communicative style and language frequently affect the outcome of clinical visits. Harmsen et al. (2003), for instance, investigated the influence of cultural differences on mutual understanding and compliance in a sample of general practice patients in The Netherlands. They found that communications in consultations between GPs and persons from ethnic minorities were less effective than consultations with Dutch persons, in that there was more misunderstanding and greater non-compliance. In line with this, research has shown the advantages of the doctor and patient speaking the same native language, in terms of greater rapport, better explanations of treatment, better understanding of instructions by patients, and greater recall and question asking by patients (Thompson, 1998).

One response to differences in language use is to use an interpreter. However, there can be problems associated with this. Family members who act as interpreters may be too embarrassed, protective or defensive when they have to air issues that they think should be kept within the family (Baylav, 1996). They may also be uncomfortable disclosing to the patient what the doctor wishes to know, and may be reluctant to convey bad news. Similarly, many patients may be too embarrassed to reveal some personal and sensitive information to family members. Wherever possible, it is better to use a professional interpreter rather than a family member. However, even here, interpreters may distort what one or other party is saying, according to their own views about what is important. Thus, healthcare professionals can never be certain how accurately their words are being translated. One important point when using interpreters is that healthcare professionals should always address their comments to the patient, even though it may be tempting to talk directly to the interpreter.

Lloyd and Bor (1996) noted that communicating with patients with different cultural backgrounds may be additionally problematic, as doctors may not want to raise cross-cultural issues. This could be for several reasons, including a fear of sounding racist or prejudiced, a feeling of inadequacy, a lack of knowledge about the culture, a fear of being misunderstood or of being rejected if suggestions are not culturally acceptable, and even uncertainty about whether the patient is actually an immigrant or not. Lloyd and Bor recommended that, when communicating with patients with different ethnic backgrounds, healthcare professionals should use open questions, explore the racial and cultural background only if necessary, and be honest about anything that may be unclear to them. In particular, they should show due respect for cultural differences. Healthcare professionals should not pretend to understand cultural patterns they are unclear about, be judgemental about cultural patterns or make assumptions about how cultural background might relate to onset of illness or outcome of treatment. An additional important point is that one should never view all those from a particular culture as a single category of people, who need to be treated in the same way. Just as when interacting with people from the same ethnic background as oneself, there will be differences owing to factors such as age, sex, level of education, socio-economic background, religious beliefs and so on.

Jehovah's Witnesses

One sub-group of the population who are recognized as creating a particular challenge for healthcare and health communication are Jehovah's Witnesses. The Witnesses are a Christian religious group founded in the late 1800s in the USA. A major, and well-publicized, issue in relation to healthcare is caused by the fact that Jehovah's Witnesses are devoutly religious people who believe that blood transfusion is forbidden by what is written in the Bible. In the past, this has led to court cases, with courts being required to make rulings. Particularly well-publicized cases have often involved parents making decisions about their young children. More recently, some doctors have been more willing to carry out surgical procedures without blood transfusion, but in some cases this is not practical and transfusion is seen to be essential. Clearly, the existence of such fundamentally different views on aspects of healthcare as important as blood transfusion places enormous pressures on medical staff, and creates considerable challenges for effective communication with patients and family members.

Communication with those with low levels of literacy, intelligence and learning ability

Despite our being in the twenty-first century, it is still the case that a significant proportion of the population are unable to read or write, have difficulty handling numerical information, have a low IQ or suffer from a learning disability. Illiteracy is particularly common in less developed countries. However, even in the Western world, millions of children still leave school without being able to read or write. A BBC news item in 2005 (BBC, 2005b) reported that one-fifth of adults in the UK have severe problems with reading and writing. A survey (BBC, 2005b) showed that 20 per cent of adults were not able to find a plumber in the *Yellow Pages* telephone directory (even though many were listed). Similar rates have been reported in recent studies in the USA, with 20 per cent of working adults reported as being illiterate or having severe difficulties reading and writing (Facts on Illiteracy in America, 2005). An even greater proportion of people have difficulties handling numerical information. Schwartz et al. (1997), for example, found that only 16 per cent of 500 women were able to answer three simple numeracy questions correctly. Similar results were reported by Lipkus et al. (2001), and by Bynner and Parsons (1997) in their study of the 1998 birth cohort.

A new and related concept that has emerged in recent years is that of health literacy. The World Health Organization defined health literacy as the cognitive and social skills which determine the motivation and ability of individuals to gain access to, understand and use information in ways which promote and maintain good health (Nutbeam, 1998). In line with this, Doak et al. (1998) described the cognitive abilities that contribute to health literacy as being verbal fluency and having the ability to understand word meanings, to scan visual information in order to identify key concepts, and to separate out key points from less relevant details, as well as being able to understand and interpret numbers. More recently, particularly with the massive growth in access to health information via the Internet, computer literacy has been included as an element of general health literacy.

In an early study in this area, Williams et al. (1995) found that a third of English speakers and nearly two-thirds of Spanish speakers in two large US hospitals were unable to complete simple reading and numeracy tasks that are necessary for effective functioning in the hospital context. They also reported that over 40 per cent of the sample was not able to understand the directions for taking their prescribed medicines correctly. These findings were confirmed in a more recent study by the Institute of Medicine in the USA. They found that nearly half of the adult population in the USA (90 million people) had health literacy levels that meant that they would have difficulty understanding and acting on health information (Davis and Wolf, 2004). The situation is not helped by the fact that much of the available information is not tailored to the needs of such people. Wallace and Lennon (2004), for instance, examined the readability of American Academy of Faculty Physicians' patient education materials available via the Internet, and found that 75 per cent of handouts were written above the average reading level of American adults.

Davis and Wolf (2004) pointed out that health literacy is increasingly being recognized as a problem that influences both healthcare quality and cost. In line with this, Bernhardt and Cameron (2003) argued that a lack of health literacy can have a significant negative effect on people's health, in that it can lead to poorer adherence, increased levels of unhealthy behaviours and adverse health outcomes, and higher healthcare costs and hospitalization rates. They went on to suggest that healthcare professionals need to look out for low-literacy warning signs when communicating with patients. These might include patients taking a long time to write their name, using surrogates for written tasks, asking if they can return paperwork at a later date, and frequently asking for information to be repeated. When interacting with such people, professionals should keep messages as clear and simple as possible, use short sentences and avoid over-reliance on medical jargon.

Repetition should be used to reinforce key points. Healthcare professionals should not revert to speaking loudly when interacting with people who have limited understanding, and should not show signs of impatience.

Uncommunicative patients

Another difficulty for health communication is that some patients are very withdrawn and difficult to engage in conversation. This may be limited to a reluctance to interact or it may also include the patient refusing to take actions, such as adhere to treatment programmes. As noted by Lloyd and Bor (1996), there may be many reasons for a patient being uncommunicative, in that they may be:

♦ particularly shy and reserved
♦ embarrassed about some aspect of their problem
♦ feeling sad or depressed
♦ experiencing considerable pain
♦ suffering from physical or cognitive impairments that affect understanding
♦ simply wanting to obstruct the course of the consultation.

In addition, they may be trying to protect themselves as they feel completely stressed or overwhelmed by the situation.

The first signs of an uncommunicative patient might include the patient looking away when being spoken to, hiding behind a book or magazine, or simply lying on a bed with his or her eyes closed. Healthcare professionals often feel helpless and/or redundant when trying to treat such patients. They nevertheless need to consider whether the problems are caused or exacerbated by something they have said or done, or by some aspect of the physical environment and, if so, try to address this. Many withdrawn or uncommunicative patients may give clues as to the underlying reasons for their state, even if they do not want openly to engage in a conversation. Patients may, for example, show explicit signs of anxiety, depression, anger, confusion or physical pain.

Lloyd and Bor (1996) recommended a number of guidelines for use when trying to interact with uncommunicative patients, as follows:

1 Be prepared to spend extra time in the consultation
2 Do not show signs of frustration or anger
3 Observe the patient carefully, particularly their non-verbal behaviour
4 Show empathy, for example, by using body language
5 Give a clear explanation of the purpose of the interview and what information is wanted
6 Use facilitatory language, and closed questions if necessary.

Duxbury (2000) suggested that different types of intervention might be appropriate when dealing with withdrawn or overly passive patients:

1 *Prescriptive*: healthcare professionals may need to prescribe a direct course of action, particularly in the early stages, and sometimes even carry out the action on behalf of the patient
2 *Cathartic*: it may be necessary to help the patient express feelings or undischarged emotions that are affecting their behaviour, so that they can be addressed more directly
3 *Catalytic*: the aim here is to bring about a return to well-being by facilitating a change in behaviour and lifestyle by helping the patient to develop and use new skills, and to grow in confidence.

Communicating with angry or aggressive patients

The final category of people, to be considered in this chapter, who pose challenges for effective health communication, are excessively angry or aggressive patients or family members. The amount of aggression and violence in healthcare encounters is reported to be increasing, with verbal abuse and minor injuries being the two most common forms (Duxbury, 2000). In some circumstances there might be understandable reasons for anger, even if the response seems overly strong. This might include situations where patients or relatives have just been given bad news, such as diagnosis of a terminal illness or death of a loved one. Anger may also be expressed if patients or family members believe that healthcare professionals have been negligent or made some error of diagnosis or treatment, or simply are withholding information. Aggressive behaviours can also be the result of extreme lack of sleep, some head injuries and intoxication owing to drugs or alcohol. In other circumstances, however, there may be no obvious reason for anger or aggression. In such cases, there may well be a history of previous aggression or abuse.

When faced with angry patients or relatives, healthcare professionals sometimes get defensive and try to explain why the anger is not justified. However, this is not advisable as it may well exacerbate the situation, which might result in the person becoming aggressive. Instead, they should invite the patient or family member to explain why they are angry, trying to remain calm and respectful while they do so. Preliminary signs of aggression include changes in speech rate and intensity, loss of eye contact and other changes in facial expression, explicit signs of impatience and trembling. There can also be changes in body language, such as closing in on the professional or using sudden expansive movements. Healthcare professionals need to learn to recognize these signs and to react appropriately when they occur.

Farrell and Gray (1992) proposed a three-stage model of aggression management:

1 Reflect – this encompasses the potential use of self in producing both therapeutic and non-therapeutic encounters

2 Relate – this involves a combination of interpersonal skills, particularly in diffusing difficult situations, and sometimes physical interventions such as resistance

3 Review – this final stage involves reviewing actions and outcomes, and is said to be vital for healing as well as learning for the future.

Following this, Lloyd and Bor (1996) outlined a number of more specific guidelines for healthcare professionals when dealing with excessively angry or aggressive patients and relatives. They suggested that professionals should:

♦ acknowledge the anger and show a willingness to talk and listen
♦ ask open rather than closed questions
♦ not interrupt or threaten patients or relatives in any way
♦ not make agreements or promises that obviously cannot be kept
♦ help the patient feel that they have choices
♦ not talk to angry or aggressive people from behind as this can be threatening and unnerving for them
♦ try not to take personal offence or get too involved emotionally
♦ keep at a safe distance if the patient is showing signs of aggression
♦ if the situation gets too threatening, summon assistance (e.g. from security staff), but try to supervise the way they deal with the situation and retain control where possible.

Summary

This chapter has looked at challenges to effective communication that are posed by healthcare providers having to interact with, and treat, various different sub-groups of the population, including older adults, young children and parents, adolescents, people with different cultural and religious backgrounds, those with low levels of literacy and intelligence, uncommunicative patients, and angry or aggressive patients and relatives. In each case, advice has been provided for how healthcare professionals might improve their communications in order to benefit patient care. This theme is continued in the next chapter, which looks at communication in difficult circumstances, such as when a healthcare professional has to convey complex information or deliver bad news.

SCHOOL OF HEALTH & SOCIAL CARE
Library
0 1 AUG 2008
Arrowe Park Site
UNIVERSITY OF CHESTER

Communication of difficult information and in difficult circumstances

Medicine and healthcare will inevitably involve the need for difficult conversations, and probably more so than in most other professions. One reason for this is that medical information is often complex and difficult to convey, such as when trying to communicate information about risk and uncertainty. Another is that healthcare professionals sometimes have to deliver particularly bad or distressing news. This chapter looks at some of the issues that arise in such circumstances and offers some suggestions to help healthcare professionals improve interactions with patients and family members. It ends by considering some of the ethical issues that arise in health communications, including those associated with truth telling and gaining fully informed consent.

Communicating information about risk and uncertainty

Medical and health-related information is often, by its very nature, complex. Evidence may be ambiguous or appear contradictory. It is often uncertain, in that not all the facts are known, as well as being dynamic and unstable, in that it changes over time as new information becomes available. In addition, many patients have multiple health problems and are treated by several different healthcare providers. Their different medical problems may have separate and interacting risks associated with them and their treatment. It has frequently been noted that communicating information about risk and uncertainty is a particularly difficult matter for healthcare professionals (e.g. Berry, 2004; Schultz, 1998). There is not only the difficulty of determining which information to convey, but also the issue of how best to present it in order to facilitate understanding and increase the likelihood of appropriate action.

Risk was defined by the British Medical Association in 1990 as 'the probability that something unpleasant will happen' (BMA, 1990, p. 14). Thus, it is not certain that the event will occur but, if it does, the event will have negative rather than positive consequences. Given that there is risk associated with almost everything we do, or that happens to us, healthcare professionals need to determine which risks are the most relevant and significant ones that need to be communicated to patients or family members. This will involve consideration of the severity of the risk (such as whether it is life threatening or not) as well as the likelihood of it occurring. It is probably not worth telling a patient about a large number of possible complications or adverse events that are very unlikely to occur and that would not have any serious consequences even if they did. In addition to considering objective severity and likelihood, it is also necessary to take account of the potential effect of a specific adverse outcome on a particular patient's experience or lifestyle. Different people attach different values to different types of risk. What may seem to be a very minor matter for one patient, or for a healthcare professional, may be a matter of considerable concern for another person. For example, in an unpublished norming study we carried out a few years ago, we asked a large number of people to rate their perceived severity of a large number of potential side effects of a medicine. We found that students rated acne as being relatively severe, whereas doctors rated it as being very mild and inconsequential.

Taking account of considerations such as these, MacDonald (2004) suggested that there are six questions that healthcare professionals need to consider when wanting to communicate risk information. These are:

1 What are the pertinent unwanted outcomes?
2 How permanent is any unwanted outcome?
3 When will the unwanted outcome occur?
4 How likely is the unwanted outcome?
5 Does this result from a single exposure or multiple exposures with cumulative risk?
6 How much does the unwanted outcome matter to this individual person?

In general, in thinking about the content of risk messages, it is clear that this needs to take account of both patient needs and healthcare providers' goals, and find an appropriate balance between these if there is any conflict. Risk information also needs to be fair and balanced. This includes giving information about treatment benefits as well as risks. As Cuervo and Aronson (2004) argued, in all areas of healthcare, we need information about all the effects, both beneficial and harmful, of relevant interventions, if patients and healthcare professionals are to take a balanced view of the therapeutic benefits and harms of treatments. In line with this, recent research has shown that the provision of information about treatment benefits can significantly affect people's satisfaction and likelihood of accepting and adhering to the treatment (e.g. Bersellini and Berry, 2004, in press). Risk communication also needs to be based on up-to-date scientific evidence, and should come from a trusted source. Even the most well constructed and presented communication will not be accepted and acted on if the recipients do not have faith in the source of the information.

In recent years, it has become increasingly apparent that there is more to effective risk communication than simply getting the content of risk messages correct (e.g. Berry 2004, 2006; Paling, 2004). The 'right' content will not necessarily bring about the desired effects, and may lead to unwanted or harmful effects, if it is not presented in an appropriate way and interpreted by the recipient in the way intended by the communicator. As we will see later, the 1995 'pill scare' in the UK was a classic example of this.

Conveying risk information is particularly challenging as we know that many people are cognitively and/or emotionally ill-equipped to understand, retain and use risk information effectively (e.g. Berry, 2004; Doyal, 2001). A large number of people have difficulties interpreting numerical information, and virtually all of us are subject to cognitive biases and are influenced by the particular way in which information is presented. Some of the most notable ways in which our understanding and behaviours are influenced by the way information is presented are described later (see also Berry, 2006).

Verbal versus numerical descriptions of risk likelihood

Healthcare providers often have to inform patients about the likelihood of particular risks occurring. This is usually done using verbal labels, such as 'common' or 'rare', or using numerical terms, such as '1 in 10' or '10 per cent'. As far as the former is concerned, there is a good deal of evidence to show that people vary considerably in their interpretation of terms that are commonly used to describe risk likelihood, even in relatively restricted domains (e.g. Bryant and Norman, 1980; Mazur and Merz, 1994: Timmermans, 1994). Bryant and Norman (1980), for example, found that physicians' interpretations of the term 'likely' ranged from 25 per cent to 75 per cent. Similarly, Timmermans (1994) reported that interpretations of the term 'very likely' ranged from 30 per cent to 90 per cent even when presented in a restricted medical context. More recently, together with co-workers, I have carried out a series of studies showing that use of verbal descriptors (such as 'common' or 'rare') recommended by the European Union for description of medication side effects on Patient Information Leaflets leads to a considerable over-estimation of risk in members of the general population, hospital patients and doctors (e.g. Berry et al., 2002, 2004; Knapp et al., 2004).

Such problems with the interpretation of verbal labels have led some researchers and practitioners to argue that risk likelihood should be conveyed using numerical terms. However, there is also considerable evidence that many people have difficulty interpreting such information (e.g. Lipkus et al., 2001; Schwarz et al., 1997; Sheridan and Pignone, 2002), particularly when presented using percentages (e.g. Gigerenzer, 2002). In terms of the latter, Hoffrage et al. (2000) found that medical students were significantly more correct on a series of medical diagnosis problems when the statistics were communicated as natural frequencies (such as 1 in 10) rather than as percentages. Even natural frequencies, however, can cause problems for some individuals, and in some circumstances, particularly when comparing two different risk likelihoods (Paling, 2004). In general, given the limitations of both forms of presentation, the safest strategy is to describe risk likelihood using common verbal descriptors together with the associated natural frequencies.

Framing effects

Another key way in which the form of presentation of risk information influences interpretations and subsequent behaviours concerns whether a message is framed positively or negatively. We are all familiar with the expression 'is the bottle half full (positive framing) or half empty (negative framing)?'. It is now well established (e.g. Gurm and Litaker, 2000; McNeil et al., 1982) that people are much more likely to opt for particular treatments, for example, if the information is framed positively (e.g. that there is a 90 per cent chance of survival) rather than negatively (e.g. that there is a 10 per cent risk of dying). Gurm and Litaker (2000), for instance, found that patients were significantly more likely to opt for angioplasty treatment when told it was '99 per cent safe' compared with there being a '1 per cent risk of a serious complication'. Framing effects are particularly prevalent in situations where people do not hold strong pre-existing beliefs about the situation.

Absolute and relative risk

In many situations, healthcare professionals often have to inform patients about risk reductions or increases. The two most commonly used methods for doing this are 'absolute risk formats' and 'relative risk formats'. Thus, a risk reduction from 6 per cent to 3 per cent can be described as an absolute risk reduction of 3 per cent or, in relative terms, as having halved or reduced by 50 per cent. It is becoming increasingly recognized that presenting risk increases or reductions as relative values can significantly bias people's understanding of the information. Malenka et al. (1993), for instance, found that nearly 80 per cent of their participants opted for the medicine that was presented with information about relative risk benefits, compared with 20 per cent for the medicine presented with information about absolute risk benefits. More recently, Hembroff et al. (2004) found that study participants were significantly less likely to recommend a medicine for preventing bone disease to a friend when the risks were described in relative as opposed to absolute terms.

Such biases can have serious consequences for health behaviours and outcomes, as shown by the 1995 'pill scare' in the UK. This was caused by the Committee on Safety of Medicines issuing a warning that third-generation oral contraceptives were associated with around twice the risk of venous thrombosis compared with second-generation pills. This warning was picked up, and dramatically reported, by the media, with the result that many women stopped taking the pill. Unfortunately, this resulted in a large number of unwanted pregnancies and terminations. What the women were not told, however, was that the absolute risk level was actually very low (and, even when doubled, was still lower than the risk of thrombosis in pregnancy). Recent studies by our research group have shown that such biased behaviour can be avoided if people are given information about the baseline (or pre-treatment) level of risk (Natter and Berry, 2005).

One might think that those trying to communicate risk information in relation to health matters would have learned from the detrimental consequences of the pill scare. However, drug companies and healthcare agencies are still presenting risks in relative terms. For example, in 2002 (seven years after the pill scare) the UK press reported research findings that hormone replacement therapy (HRT) had been found to cause a 26 per cent increase in risk of breast cancer, a 41 per cent increase in risk of stroke and a 29 per cent increase in risk of heart attack. Again, there was no reference to the absolute levels of risk involved. In reality, the risk of breast cancer as a result of HRT for a five-year period is estimated at '4 women per 1000', that is (as noted by Paling, 2004) 996 women will be safe!

The order of information

Healthcare professionals should not only consider the format in which to present information, but they should also think about the order of information, as this can affect people's understanding and memory of the information. A study by my research group (Berry et al., 1998) presented people with a simplified medicines information leaflet and found that, in order to be remembered, information about drug administration (for example, dosage and how to take the medicine) had to be given near to the start of the leaflet. In contrast, information about adverse side effects was well remembered irrespective of its relative position. It is likely that this order effect is related to the perceived importance of the information. Subjective ratings showed that information about side effects was rated as being much more important than information about drug administration. Healthcare professionals should therefore present key information, particularly that which patients might not believe to be important, near to the start of risk messages.

Genetic counselling

Helping patients and families to understand risks is a fundamental part of genetic counselling. There has been a massive increase in the use of genetic counselling in recent years and this trend is set to continue. Tests already exist for nearly 500 conditions and, with advances in scientific knowledge of the human genome, this number will increase significantly in the coming years. Our ability to predict an increased likelihood of developing certain diseases imposes some profound ethical questions and raises some practical problems for patients, genetic counsellors, doctors and wider society (Loewy and Loewy, 2004). Effective communication between all parties is vital, given the potential difficulties involved. As noted by Loewy and Loewy (2004), the language we use when communicating genetic information can be crucial to how information is understood and accepted. In genetics, the question of what is considered to be 'normal', and how this is defined and conveyed, will affect people's perception of genetic information and their resulting behaviour. Thus, for example, acceptance (or otherwise) of therapeutic abortion will depend on what one considers to be a 'normal' foetus. There may well be different perspectives on this, however, depending on who is doing the accepting.

There are relatively few empirical studies that have looked at communication and information giving in genetic counselling settings. Lobb et al. (2004) recently carried out a longitudinal study to do this, with women from familial breast cancer families. The study documented information giving and patient communication styles of counsellors in familial breast cancer clinics, and assessed their effects on women's knowledge, expectations, satisfaction, risk perception and psychological status. They found that discussing genetic testing significantly decreased anxiety and depression. In addition, receiving a summary letter following the consultation also led to reduced anxiety and increased accuracy of risk perception.

Conveying information about the outcome of genetic tests often poses ethical dilemmas for the healthcare professionals concerned. In some situations, patients may decide against what the professionals believe is the right course of action. When such decisions only impact on the patient him- or herself, the professionals might find this easier to accept. However, when there are potentially serious implications for others, as is often the case with genetic information, healthcare professionals are likely to experience some form of divided loyalty. Thus, for example, a patient might refuse the offer of a therapeutic abortion, even when the baby would be profoundly disabled and be likely to have an extremely poor quality of life. Similarly, a patient might be given the results of a genetic test that should be shared with certain other family members (as they too may be affected by the condition), but the patient refuses for the information to be divulged to the relatives concerned. The question of addressing ethical issues such as these will be returned to later in this chapter.

In many situations, genetic counsellors and other healthcare professionals will have to convey potentially distressing news to patients. The next section of this chapter looks more closely at the problems associated with conveying bad news in healthcare.

Conveying bad news

The practice of medicine and healthcare inevitably involves healthcare professionals having to break bad news to patients and family members. The scale of this will range from informing a patient that they may need an operation, which is likely to disrupt their work and lifestyle in some way, through to informing them of a terminal diagnosis, or informing relatives of an unexpected death. In all cases, the need for good communication skills is essential. Healthcare professionals need to be able to take account of the recipient's state and likely response throughout the discussion, and adjust their style, and pace of imparting information, to take account of this. Most people need time to absorb key information in such circumstances, and to come to terms with the likely implications.

Ptacek and Eberhardt (1996) carried out a review of 67 selected studies on 'breaking bad news' and came up with the following key recommendations:

1 Choose a quiet, comfortable and private location
2 Choose a convenient time, if possible, that will ensure that there are no interruptions and that sufficient time is available
3 Sit close to the person and engage in direct eye contact
4 Start the communication with some preparatory statement. Use this to find out what the patient knows and how they are likely to react
5 Allow time for, and encourage, questions and summarize key points at the end of the discussion
6 Use warmth, care, empathy and respect
7 Adopt a simple and direct language, avoiding medical jargon where possible, and avoiding euphemisms
8 Impart the news at the patient's pace, not the healthcare professional's.

In line with this, Lloyd and Bor (1996) recommended that breaking bad news requires empathy, starting with what the patient already knows and understands, and finding out what they want to know. It also involves active listening and giving information, eliciting the patient's own resources for coping, and instilling realistic hope. In addition, it is important to let the patient or relatives know what the next steps will be.

Clearly, healthcare professionals will often find delivering bad news to be a stressful event. This may be because they feel responsible in some way or fear being blamed. It may also be because they do not know the patient or family member very well, or that they simply do not know how best to deliver the news. Whatever the reason, healthcare professionals should not delay imparting the news for any longer than is necessary or reasonable. In some circumstances, it may be helpful to include other healthcare providers in the discussions. For example, a doctor might want to involve one or more nurses who are much more familiar with the patient than he or she is, when conveying difficult news to patients or family members.

From the patient perspective, they may also prefer to have one or more family members present when being given distressing news, although this is not always the case. The presence of significant others may be particularly beneficial if the patient has difficulty taking in all the key information, as it will give them more opportunity for further informed discussion once they have left the consultation. As noted by MacDonald (2004), an important point is to try to leave the patient, and/or family, with some 'degree of hope' at the end of the discussion. Even if the prognosis is terminal, patients must still be reassured about pain management and maintenance of comfort and dignity. However, it is essential not to give false hope. Patients or relatives may attach far too much importance to any statement that gives even the remotest glimmer of hope. Replacement of words such as 'death' or 'dying' with euphemisms can result in patients not registering the enormity of the situation, and therefore should be avoided.

Communication with dying patients

Having to deliver news of a terminal diagnosis, and ongoing communications with patients and family members as an illness progresses to its final stages, can be particularly demanding for healthcare professionals. Curtis et al. (2001), for example, emphasized that communication with cancer patients and their families during the end-of-life process is probably one of the most challenging aspects of cancer care for all concerned. Some professionals react to the situation by trying to avoid communication. However, cutting off communication at a time a patient probably needs it most is neglecting a key part of caring for the patient. As stressed by Fletcher (1980, 1988), no news is not good news, it is an invitation to fear.

In general, it is not *if*, but *how*, the truth should be told that is the issue (Loewy and Loewy, 2004). Patients need to be gently led to receive news of a terminal diagnosis. The emphasis should be on human understanding, rather than on conveying technical knowledge. As Loewy and Loewy (2004) noted, 'talking to patients who must be given news that they are hopelessly ill truly requires compassionate rationality' (p. 292). Health professionals need to show compassion but they must remain rational and not become too emotionally involved.

Research has shown that the quality of communication throughout the end-of-life process is critical to providing effective care for patients who are dying (Larson and Tobin, 2000). The emphasis of communication in word, attitude and behaviour, needs to convey the message that 'the patient is safe and treasured as an individual in their own right' (MacDonald, 2004, p. 62). Patients (and their loved ones) need reassurance that death will be dignified, comfortable and caring.

Kubler-Ross (1969) outlined five stages through which patients with a progressive fatal illness generally pass. These are: denial, anger, bargaining, depression and, finally, acceptance. During the first stage, many patients try to convince themselves that the diagnosis and test information are wrong. Following this, when they accept the truth, some express anger, questioning why the situation has happened to them. In the bargaining stage, patients might try to be rewarded for good behaviour, even though this is futile. Once they realize this, then depression can set in before full acceptance finally occurs. Clearly, not all patients will go through all of the stages. However, it is useful to bear the different states in mind when attempting to communicate with patients during the end-of-life process.

As an illness progresses, some patients may want to make advance directives that stipulate what should be done if they lose their capacity to make decisions and communicate these to healthcare professionals. Given that patients may not be able to foresee how their illness will progress, it is recommended that they seek medical advice when drawing up any directives. Once made, it is important that patients know that their future wishes will be respected, provided that the directives are legally enforceable demands.

Communication issues in the treatment and care of cancer patients

Much of the research on breaking bad news and communicating with people who are terminally ill has been carried out in the area of cancer. As noted by Kreps (2003), cancer is a complex array of different kinds of health challenges, with many different sites, stages, causes, screening strategies, treatment strategies and responses to treatment. A large amount of complex, and changing, information needs to be communicated to different individuals, who vary in terms of their needs, cognitive abilities and emotional state. To make matters more difficult, cancer information is often highly emotionally charged, owing to associations with pain, suffering and death. Thus, cancer poses a series of health threats that demand effective health communication (Kreps, 2003). We know that effective communication with patients and families, that appropriately co-ordinates both the content and relational aspects of the process, is central to the quality of cancer care, from primary prevention to survivorship or end-of-life care. As Kreps (2003) pointed out, effective health communication has a great potential to help reduce cancer risks, incidence, morbidity and mortality, while enhancing quality of life across the continuum of cancer care (prevention, detection, diagnosis, treatment, survivorship and end-of-life care). Thus, for example, communication is the primary process for promoting cancer prevention through information campaigns, as well being the key way of informing and motivating people to seek screening for early detection of cancer.

Although communication is also a vital part of treating and caring for cancer patients, studies have shown that the process is not always carried out smoothly and effectively. Thus, as noted by Fallowfield (2002), consultations with patients and their families about cancer pose many difficulties owing to the need to convey difficult information about aspects of treatment and care (such as explaining complex treatment options and the need for clinical trials), obtaining informed consent, informing people about diagnoses of recurrence and discussing transition from active therapy to palliative care. Not surprisingly, both patients and health professionals experience problems with much of this communication (Fallowfield, 2002). In line with this, studies have shown that cancer patients and their families often have many unmet information needs. Interestingly, research has also shown that failure to discuss issues of most concern to patients and their relatives sometimes stems from a lack of awareness, but more often arises because 'talking about cancer and its treatment can be very difficult and emotionally taxing for patients and doctors' (Fallowfield, 2002, p. 80).

A number of factors contribute to the difficulties that are experienced by the different parties involved. For example, diagnoses of cancer often occur in a busy hospital setting, are given in a disjointed fashion, and take place on wards and in corridors, over a series of days or even weeks as information becomes available (e.g. Schou and Hewison, 1999). It is not unusual for diagnostic experiences to involve several health professionals, different hospital departments, many tests, exploratory surgery and time waiting for test results to become available. As noted by Schou and Hewison (1999), diagnoses (including attendant prognostic, treatment rationale and follow-up information) are often not so much given by clinicians to patients, as they are revealed (usually partially) by clinicians and interpreted by patients. Studies have shown that some patients have not actually been given an explicit diagnosis of cancer. Thus, Schou and Hewison reported a patient being told by a surgeon that the suspicions of the referring consultant had been confirmed, but there was no acknowledgement of what these suspicions were (that is, cancer was not mentioned). They also noted that it is not unusual for patients, or their GPs, to receive letters about starting radiotherapy treatment before being told that they actually had cancer. Although, in practice, most patients do now receive their diagnosis, fewer of them are informed about their prognosis. Unfortunately, these issues do not just apply to patients with cancer; they are also common in other terminal illnesses.

Research has also shown that difficulties arise because patients and health professionals often have very different perspectives on the information needs of patients and their families. Treatment professionals are often primarily concerned with treatment, whereas the cause of the illness tends to be a key issue for patients, so that they can place the cancer in context and make appropriate lifestyle changes. Similarly, continuity of care (for example, always seeing the same doctor) is an important aspect for patients, while doctors see it as a much lower priority for doctors (Van der Waal et al., 1996). One reason for these differences, and for many of the difficulties involved in communication in cancer care, is that most health professionals have not received adequate training in communication skills. In line with this, many oncologists acknowledge that insufficient communication skills training is a major contributory factor to their stress, lack of job satisfaction and burnout (Fallowfield, 2002). As we will see in Chapter 8, effective training in communication skills can significantly improve the quality of patient treatment and care.

Withdrawal of active treatment / life support

Many patients, relatives and even doctors may find it difficult to accept that there can come a time when active treatment is no longer likely to be of any benefit to the patient. It is important to explain, however, that this does not mean that the patient will no longer be given any treatment. Rather, treatment will focus on the relief of symptoms, and maintenance of comfort and dignity, as opposed to prolonging life. When communicating with patients and relatives, it is essential that healthcare professionals explain that the aim of treatment may change but the quality of care will not. MacDonald (2004) suggested that it may be useful to remind patients and relatives of the patient's history, the seriousness of his or her condition, and what treatments have been tried and were not, or are no longer, helping the patient. In addition, people should be informed about what will happen from now on and who will be responsible for care of the patient in the next stages of the illness. One key point that MacDonald stressed is that healthcare providers should never use the phrase 'nothing more can be done', as this has a desperate ring and may leave people feeling abandoned and helpless.

One situation where withdrawal of active treatment may be likely to occur is in intensive care units. In such cases, direct communication is not usually possible and it is often necessary to carry out critical discussions with relatives. The decision to withdraw life support is a matter for the healthcare professionals treating the patient rather than for the family members themselves, although, of course, the latter will be consulted. Legally, relatives are not in a position to refuse treatment on behalf of another adult, unless legal provision has been made for this. When communicating the decision to withdraw life support, healthcare professionals need to explain that continuation of support is futile as it would simply be prolonging the 'dying period' rather than maintaining life. Again, however, there is a need to stress that there will be no withdrawal of 'treatment for comfort'.

Breaking news of unexpected death

In many circumstances, the death of a patient is not unexpected as relatives may be aware of the seriousness of a patient's condition and the likely prognosis. However, there are other occasions when people die unexpectedly, such as following a major heart attack or stroke, or as the result of an accident. Breaking news of unexpected death is clearly very challenging for healthcare professionals as family members are likely to be in a state of shock when they are informed of the death. It is often the case that the healthcare professional involved will not know the patient or their relatives. As with all serious conversations in healthcare, it is important that the news is broken in a private, quiet location, and in a calm and sympathetic manner. The family member, or members, present need to be given time to assimilate what they are being told, and repetition of key facts may be necessary. One issue that can arise in the case of a sudden, unexpected death is that the medical team may not have all of the answers to the relatives' questions, as they may not know at that time exactly what has caused the death. In some cases it is necessary for a post-mortem to be carried out before the cause is established. It is difficult to predict how families will react to the news of an unexpected death. Some want to have an extended discussion, trying to elicit information and gain a full understanding of what has occurred. Others simply want to get away from the bearer of the bad news in order to be on their own. It is important in both circumstances, however, that relatives are offered some form of support.

It is often that case that family members will want to have a subsequent discussion with the healthcare team who treated the patient or who were present at the time of death. Many relatives will find comfort in talking to such staff about the events surrounding the death. However, healthcare professionals may feel difficult in such situations and may feel that their time would be better spent helping those who still have a chance of survival rather than talking to the bereaved. It is important that healthcare providers do talk to bereaved relatives, at least until all of the essential information has been conveyed. After this, they need to direct the family towards other sources of support for the bereaved.

Another difficult communication issue that arises in both intensive care and in the case of sudden death is that it is the duty of doctors to ask about organ donation if this is appropriate (see also Sque and Payne, in press). If the patient is a registered donor then the situation may be more straightforward but, in either case, the family still has to make the decision as to whether or not organs can be donated. Studies have shown that where the patient's wishes are not known, around 50 to 70 per cent of families will agree to donation (MacDonald, 2004). It is important that the healthcare professional who makes the request is comfortable with the idea of donation. Interestingly, Gross et al. (2000) reported that 23 per cent of healthcare staff in a community hospital in Switzerland would not agree to a close relative's organs being donated if the patient's wishes were not known in advance. Studies have shown that the likelihood of relatives agreeing to organ donation is increased if the request is decoupled from patient care (that is, if brainstem death has already been accepted), if the request is made in a quiet, private room and if a transplant co-ordinator is involved (Gortmaker et al., 1998). Agreement is also more likely if families are satisfied with the hospital care that their relatives have received (De Jong et al., 1998). In addition, it can be helpful for healthcare professionals to suggest that out of their tragedy, there could be a benefit for some other family.

Admitting to errors and making apologies

Given the complexity of clinical medicine and the pressures on healthcare staff, it is almost inevitable that errors will occasionally be made. It is important that, when errors are discovered, patients and/or their families are informed as soon as possible, and preferably by a senior member of the healthcare team. As pointed out by MacDonald (2004), people need to be advised about the exact nature and scale of the error, and the likely consequences. They also need to be told how the error came about and what can be done to reduce the likelihood of future errors. Patients and family members will be keen to know that lessons have been learned for the future. They may well want a full investigation of the circumstances and will often feel and express anger. As usual in such difficult circumstances, it is important that healthcare professionals allow sufficient time for discussions and attempt to answer all of the patient's or relatives' questions. It can be helpful for the healthcare professional involved to express regret that an error has been made. However, disclosing an error and expressing regret is not the same thing as accepting that negligence or liability has occurred (MacDonald, 2004). It is important that, when apologies are made, the professional concerned does not say anything that would commit his or her employers to any legal liability.

Ethical issues in health communication

Much of the emphasis in this book so far has concerned the need for, and benefit of, effective health communications. However, in addition to being effective, communication must also be ethical. Beauchamp and Childress (1994) outlined four basic principles that are central to medical ethics. These are as follows:

1 *Respect for patient autonomy*. Autonomy is the right of individuals to decide for themselves what they want to do. Thus, respect for autonomy requires health professionals to help patients to make their own decisions,

and to respect these, even if they disagree with the patients' wishes. Schneider (1998) distinguished between two different types of autonomy: the optional model and the mandatory model. Basically, according to the former model, a patient is entitled, but not required, to take an active role in decision making. In contrast, the mandatory model holds that people need to exercise their autonomy and must do so.

2 *Beneficence*. This principle is concerned with the notion of benefiting patients, and it involves health professionals doing their best to act on behalf of patients. In many situations, acting in line with this principle will have the same outcome as will respecting patient autonomy. As we will see later, however, there can be a conflict between the two, when healthcare providers believe that following the patient's wishes will not result in optimal health outcomes.

3 *Non-maleficence*. This principle states that health professionals should not harm their patients. It has its roots in the Hippocratic oath that physicians have to take, but that other healthcare providers also try to follow. The oath declares that physicians will dedicate themselves to helping the sick and to doing them no harm. It is therefore also closely related to the principle of beneficence. Clearly, many health interventions will carry some degree of risk. This does not mean that they must therefore be avoided. Rather, it is up to the healthcare team to weigh the level of harm against the potential benefits, when determining the best course of action.

4 *Justice*. The final principle requires health professionals to be fair to patients. It requires their treating patients who are in similar situations equally. This principle is receiving increasing attention, as people are living longer, technology is advancing (and resulting treatments are often more costly), and resources are essentially limited. In recent years in the UK, there have been several well-publicized legal cases where patients have brought action about local health authorities for withholding costly medical treatments that they feel should be available to them. As noted by Danis and Churchill (1991), in a situation of limited resources, the needs of both the individual and the public cannot always be met simultaneously.

Morgan and Lave (1990) distinguished between ethical issues that arise at the individual level and those that arise at the institutional or society level. Health professionals frequently have to address the former as part of their day-to-day work. For example, doctors and other healthcare professionals are often faced with decisions about how much information to give patients about their condition, the risks of potential treatments, the results and implications of genetic tests, and so on. Similar issues arise in relation to screening. For example, in pre-implantation screening, one can ask the question, whose interests are paramount – the embryo's or the future parents (Markham, 1998)? Screening can also raise ethical issues at the societal level. Thus, for example, should a less effective procedure for a relatively common condition take priority (when resources are limited) over a very effective procedure for a much rarer condition? To date, policy makers have tended to make such choices by adopting the principle of 'the greatest good for the greatest number of people'.

Parker (2004) identified four main challenges to ethical communication. The first is where patients (in the view of the health professional) make the 'wrong' treatment choice (see also Parker et al., 2004). Thus, for example, a patient might be given a choice between two potential treatments; one being more effective but involving more temporary adverse side effects, and the second being much less effective but not involving the adverse effects. The patient might opt for the latter, whereas the health professional would strongly recommend the former. In such cases, should the healthcare provider try to bias patients by presenting the key information in a particular way, or try to encourage them to change their minds by making it clear what they would do in the same situation? The second challenge is where health professionals believe that patients have made the 'wrong' moral choice. This situation could arise, for example, when a patient is given the result of a genetic test that should be shared with family members who might be affected, but chooses not to do so. Would it ever be right for the health professional concerned to inform the relatives of the test result themselves? The third challenge identified by Parker is where patients want no information at all about their illness or potential treatments. Research has shown that patients vary in their information needs and demands. Thus, those who are more elderly or who are more seriously ill tend to want less information, and be less involved in decision making about their care, than those who are younger or less seriously ill (e.g. Ryan, 1992). However, healthcare professionals can be faced with patients who want no information at all about their condition or its treatment. They simply want the doctor, or other healthcare providers involved, to make the necessary decisions and take the necessary actions on their behalf. As we will see shortly, this raises considerable issues when trying to respect the need to gain 'fully informed consent'. The final challenge outlined by Parker (2004) is patients who refuse life-saving treatments. In such circumstances, healthcare professionals must ensure that patients are competent to make such a choice, and that the choice is both informed and voluntary. Such matters are not always clear-cut, however, and this situation can pose considerable ethical dilemmas for healthcare providers.

Two areas of health communication that raise particular ethical issues are 'honesty' or truth telling by health professionals, and gaining informed consent. These are considered in a little more detail now.

Honesty and truth telling

As noted by Northouse and Northouse (1998), honesty and truth telling play an instrumental role in achieving ethical outcomes in healthcare. The formation and maintenance of effective interpersonal relationships between healthcare providers, patients and family members depends on honesty and trust. Patients and relatives will not develop trust in doctors and other professionals if they believe that they are not being fully honest with them. At one time it was relatively common practice for doctors (and sometimes family members) to withhold critical information from patients, particularly in the case of life-threatening diseases such as cancer. Even in the early 1990s, studies showed that some doctors were still routinely withholding key diagnostic and prognostic information from cancer sufferers. Prigerson's (1992) study, for example, found that almost half of the doctors who expected a patient to die within six months did not inform the patient of the prognosis. Even nowadays, although the norm is to be as open with patients as possible (unless the patient makes it very clear that they do not want to be given the relevant information) day-to-day practice will, and does, vary. Studies have shown that health-care providers and patients often hold different beliefs about how much information should be given to patients. Jenkins, Fallowfield and Saul (2001), for example, carried out a large survey of cancer clinics in the UK and found that doctors believed that 30 to 40 per cent of patients would not want to be given full information. However, 87 per cent of the patients said that they would want as much information as possible. In fact, only 2 per cent of 2500 patients said that they would prefer not to be given bad news.

Clearly, telling the truth comes in 'many shades and gradations' (Loewy and Loewy, 2004, p. 291). In practice, patients can only be told what they are ready to hear. Northouse and Northouse (1998) identified four different approaches to truth telling: strict paternalism, benevolent deception, con-tractual honesty and unmitigated honesty. The first approach is where the health professional blatantly lies to the patient for the presumed well-being of the patient, whereas benevolent deception involves the professional giv-ing some accurate information but also withholding some truth. Con-tractual honesty occurs where the healthcare professional provides the patient with as much information as he or she wants, whereas unmitigated honesty involves the healthcare provider giving the patient 'the whole truth' even if the patient might not want to hear it. Northouse and Northouse suggested that of the four types of honesty, contractual honesty is probably the most preferable as it respects the patient's autonomy, but, unlike unmitigated honesty, does not override their information preferences.

Informed consent

Giving patients full and honest information is a central aspect of gaining fully informed consent. From a legal point of view, informed consent involves ensuring that the patient is properly informed, has the legal capacity to give consent and does so voluntarily. The absolute legal standards of disclosure vary in different jurisdictions with, for example, the legal standard in the UK being weaker than in the USA. Generally, however, elements to be disclosed when obtaining consent include the reasons for and the nature of the benefits, risks and discomforts of the proposed treatment, the alternatives to the treatment (with comparative success rates) and the consequences of not having the treatment.

Whatever the legal position, it is the health provider's obligation to give sufficient information for truly informed decision making, not just consent. Moreover, the ethical principle of respect for a person's autonomy requires not only that patients are provided with the information, but also that they understand it. The General Medical Council in the UK has stated that patients 'must be given sufficient information, in a way that they can understand, in order to enable them to make informed decisions about their care' (GMC, 1999, p. 1). Information must be pitched not simply at what physicians would consider it necessary to disclose, but at what a reasonable person in the patient's position would find material to know. This applies not only in treatment settings, but also where patients are asked to participate in clinical trials.

Unfortunately, whether in treatment or research settings, although healthcare providers now routinely meet the legal standards in terms of information provision, relatively few meet the requirement of ensuring that patients understand the necessary information. Loewy and Loewy (2004) observed that the way consent is obtained in clinical practice is often a caricature of both informing and consenting, in that healthcare providers rarely make sure that information is truly understood. In a study of consent in a general surgery ward, Meredith (1993) found that over two-thirds of patients had not had the consent form explained to them, and over half did not know the status of the doctor requesting the signature. It emerged that house officers were often obtaining consent but were not familiar with details of treatment plans. Similarly, in relation to clinical trials, Edwards et al. (1998), when reviewing the ethics of randomized control trials, concluded that, 'doctors seemed to have been aware that patients may not have fully understood what was going on. For many, informed consent seemed little more than a ritual' (p. 1212). They reported that at an 'astonishing' 47 per cent of responding doctors in a multinational study thought that few patients knew that they were taking part in a controlled experiment, even though they had given written consent.

The failure of healthcare providers to secure patient understanding in these contexts is not altogether surprising, given that clinical information is often complex and that most people are not well equipped, either cognitively or emotionally, to interpret it effectively. As mentioned earlier, clinical information is often ambiguous, incomplete, uncertain and unstable. Moreover, many patients have multiple illnesses, with different interacting risks, and are treated by several doctors. As a result, many studies have shown that the level of patient understanding when making informed consent decisions is often fairly limited (e.g. Cassileth et al., 1980; Joffe et al., 2001). Cassileth et al. (1980), for example, interviewed 200 cancer patients undergoing chemotherapy, and found that less than half could correctly recall the purpose of their treatment one day after they had given consent. One factor that contributes to patients' lack of understanding is that much consent documentation and information is aimed more at protecting the healthcare professional and their organization than at genuinely informing the patient. Dean Acheson, an American politician in the 1930s and 1940s, once stated that 'a memorandum is written not to inform the reader but to protect the writer' (Chrystal, 2005, p. 1). Unfortunately, the same sentiment applies in relation to many informed consent materials.

It should not be surprising that the process of seeking informed consent presents doctors and other health professionals with difficult ethical issues. Different patients have different needs, wishes and cognitive abilities, so knowing how much information to give, and how best to give it, can be a problem. This is a particular issue when determining how much information to give about the risks of particular treatment options. Clearly it is not practical to inform patients about every single risk that might be involved. The legal solution to this difficulty is that patients must be informed about 'material' risks, that is, the risks that a reasonable person would wish to know in order to make an appropriate decision (Feld, 2004). However, the decision as to whether or not a risk is material is not necessarily straightforward and often 'requires the healthcare provider, in a sense, to second guess the patient' (Schultz, 1998, p. 7). Doctors often have to walk a fine line between providing pertinent risk information and not overwhelming the patient with frightening statistics (Berg et al., 2001). The situation is made more complicated as many people are cognitively and/or emotionally ill-equipped to understand, retain and use risk information effectively (Berry, 2004). The existence of such limitations, however, does not justify paying only lip-service to the goal of seeking fully informed consent. As Doyal (2001) stressed, the fact that many patients have cognitive and emotional limitations that restrict their understanding of clinical information should not undermine their potential to provide informed consent. Constraints are not convincing either moral or empirical justifications for questioning the pursuit of informed consent in clinical care.

As will be apparent from earlier in this chapter, it is virtually impossible to present completely 'neutral' risk (and benefit) information in consent documentation. An important ethical question is therefore whether there are ever any legitimate circumstances where healthcare providers should take advantage of this fact and deliberately manipulate, or hold back, information in order to increase the likelihood of consent. A distinction made in this context is one between 'informed consent' and 'informed choice'. Thus, Dickens and Cook (2004) argued that the words 'informed consent' incorrectly suggest that:

   i. patients who decide not to consent to the recommended treatment have not been properly informed

  ii. the purpose of providing information is to gain consent

 iii. patients who oppose on principle medically indicated options need not be as informed, or well informed, of consequential risks, as those not so opposed. (p. 310)

They therefore proposed that the term should be replaced with the concept 'informed choice', since the choice not to consent is 'essential to the integrated concept of voluntary or freely given consent' (p. 310).

Traditionally, when patients consent to a treatment their judgement is rarely questioned by healthcare providers but, when they do not consent, their intelligence or sanity are often called into question. However, as Loewy and Loewy (2004) noted, consent that is too glibly given should also be questioned. Patients may not have understood all the relevant information or may be frightened into assent. When a patient refuses to consent to a potentially life-saving treatment, healthcare professionals need to ensure that their choice is fully informed. This means that the patient must have understood the diagnosis, prognosis (with and without treatment), the treatment, alternatives to treatment, and that the patient is thinking clearly and is capable of giving consent or otherwise.

But are there circumstances where the freedom to choose not to consent should be questioned, even if the patient has understood the relevant information and is capable of providing consent? What about emergency, life or death situations where consent is being sought from someone other than the patient (such as carers or parents)? What about situations where there is a need to weigh up individual risks and benefits against those of other individuals or of the wider public? There can be a tension between what seems to be appropriate for an individual and what is better in the longer term for the general population. In some circumstances, greater information (e.g. about the risks of particular vaccines) could lead to informed dissent, which could then impact negatively on public health. This matter is returned to in the next chapter, where we look at communicating with the wider public. Clearly, at present, there are no clear-cut answers to issues such as these. When faced with them, healthcare professionals will have to use their own judgement in determining what action is appropriate in the given circumstances. One thing that is certain is that the number of ethical issues in relation to informed consent, and in healthcare more generally, will increase in future years as we see more and more advances in medical science and technology.

Summary

This chapter has considered a number of situations where difficult information has to be communicated to patients and/or their family members. The early part of the chapter looked at problems associated with communicating information about risk and uncertainty, and suggested some practical ways in which healthcare providers can improve their presentation of such information. The second part of the chapter focused on problems associated with delivering bad news, and looked particularly at the area of cancer. The final part of the chapter looked at the inevitable ethical issues associated with communicating difficult medical and health information. In Chapter 8 we will see that some of the difficulties associated with communicating difficult information can be addressed through effective communication skills training. Before this, we will look at health communication that occurs at the wider public health level when trying to promote better public health.

Health promotion and communicating with the wider public

Most of this book so far has focused on communication that occurs between individuals (be they healthcare professionals, patients, or relatives), or in small groups. A considerable amount of health communication, however, takes place at a wider public health, or mass communication, level. Indeed, it has been argued that the most significant determinant of health is social and economic circumstance, and that the least important is individual health behaviour (e.g. French and Adams, 2002). Thus, it has been recommended that we should focus more effort on broader public health campaigns than on trying to influence behaviour at the individual level, and that health promotion initiatives targeted at large populations are probably the most cost-effective approach to improving health (Bennett and Murphy, 1997). In a similar vein, McCormick (1996) made the case for the importance of effective health promotion by warning that if a doctor advises or treats a patient in ways that are ineffective or harmful, only that patient suffers. However, if a public health policy is ineffective or harmful, whole populations can run the risk of diminished health.

The recognition that our health depends on our environmental, social and economic circumstances is not a recent one. By the end of the nineteenth century, several studies had identified cause-and-effect relationships between things people did, or let happen, and the adverse health effects which could result. Linkages were made, for instance, between the following:

1 London smoke and respiratory disease
2 Sexual behaviour and cervical cancer
3 Tobacco snuff and cancer of the lining of the nose
4 Sunlight and skin cancer
5 Aromatic amines and cancer of the bladder
6 Contaminated water and cholera.

Clearly, in order to make linkages such as these, and to deal with problems effectively, it was, and is, necessary to address the health of the public rather than just of individuals on a one-to-one basis.

There is now clear evidence that our health status does not simply depend on biological factors but is also influenced by social, economic and psychological processes, such as diet, social class, gender, ethnicity and psychological stress. In addition, however, there are significant interactions between the different influences. Low socio-economic status, for example, can result in a lack of freedom to address environmental stressors or to engage in health-promoting behaviours. As John Reid, UK Health Minister, noted in his introduction to the UK government's White Paper on public health, that was published at the end of 2004, 'it is a fact of life that it is easier for some people to make healthy choices than others' (Department of Health, 2004, p. 2). Clearly, the existence of interactions such as these requires effective health promotion campaigns that apply multilevel interventions focused on individuals, societal, environmental and cultural processes (Bennett and Murphy, 1997).

In general, health promotion is any event, process or activity that facilitates the protection or improvement of the health status of individuals, groups, communities or populations (Marks et al., 2000). Its main objectives are to prolong life or to improve the quality of life. As Bennett and Murphy (1997) pointed out, health promotion is premised on the understanding that the behaviours in which we engage, and the circumstances in which we live, impact on our health. Health outcomes that are relevant to health promotion are increasingly recognized to result from a complex interaction between biological, social, environmental and psychological factors. In line with this, the World Health Organization (WHO) has identified the need for a multiple approach to health promotion which acknowledges the important role that the environment and public policy play in relation to health. The emphasis is more on thinking about the positive aspects of health, rather than thinking of it as the absence of disease and infirmity.

Tones (1998, pp. 1337–8) outlined five basic principles that can be used to summarize the World Health Organization's position:

- ◆ health is a positive state: quality of life and not merely quantity is important. It is an essential commodity which people need in order to achieve a socially and economically productive life
- ◆ equity should be the most important concern of health promotion: progress towards the achievement of health for all will depend on the extent to which inequalities in health within and between nations can be addressed
- ◆ health is not merely an individual responsibility: it is unethical to seek to cajole individuals into adopting healthy habits while at the same time failing to take account of the social and structural determinants of health

♦ since substantial policy change typically involves a major challenge to existing power bases, health promotion is essentially a political activity: health promotion must therefore generate political consciousness; it must mobilize communities if it is to take place as a significant part of the New Public Health movement

♦ health is too important to be left to medical professionals and so medical services must be redefined and reoriented.

In line with the WHO position, governments in the western world have been increasingly concerned about public health, and the increasing cost of 'poor public health'. Thus, many governments have set out targets for improved health, such as reducing the amount of obesity, cancer and coronary heart disease. In the UK, for example, the Department of Health published a White Paper – *Saving Lives: Our Healthier Nation* (1999) – that set out four such targets:

1 To reduce deaths from cancer by at least one-fifth (saving 100 000 lives) in people under the age of 75
2 To reduce deaths from coronary heart disease and stroke by at least two-fifths (saving 200 000 lives) in people under the age of 75
3 To reduce the number of deaths as a result of accidents by at least one-fifth (saving 12 000 lives) and reducing serious injuries by at least one-tenth
4 To reduce deaths from suicide and other mental health-related problems by at least one-fifth (saving 4000 lives).

The more recent White Paper on public health confirmed that the government's priorities for action in the coming five years would be to:

♦ reduce the numbers of people who smoke
♦ reduce obesity and improve diet and nutrition
♦ increase exercise
♦ encourage and support sensible drinking
♦ improve sexual health
♦ improve mental health (Department of Health, 2004).

In order to achieve these objectives, the UK government has committed considerable resources to fund additional posts and a new research initiative in public health, as well as improved training for existing NHS staff. They have also developed strategies for improving health via schools and the workplace. This increased emphasis on public health and health promotion is paralleled in most other countries in the western world. By the end of 1999, for example, the majority of developed countries were signed up to the WHO concept of Health Promoting Schools (Tones and Tilford, 2001).

Health promotion in schools

Rutter et al. (1979) estimated that in countries where children routinely attend school from the ages of 5 to 16, around 15 000 hours are spent there by each child. Given that this is a time when people are forming key attitudes and adopting behaviours that may last for life, it is not surprising that schools have been increasingly targeted as a focus for health education and promotion. This position was endorsed by the WHO in 1997 when they proposed that school health promotion programmes that co-ordinate the delivery of education and health services, and promote a healthy environment, could become one of the most efficient means available for almost every nation in the world to improve significantly the well-being of its people (Tones and Tilford, 2001; WHO, 1997).

Following this, the UK government published a White Paper − *Saving Lives: Our Healthier Nation* (Department of Health, 1999) − that defined a healthy school as one where good health and social behaviour underpin effective learning and academic achievement. Tones (1999) outlined the following three key elements of health-promoting schools:

1 Enhanced education for health through the formal curriculum
2 Improvements in the physical and social environment for pupils and staff to work in, including attention to how the organization of the school encourages or inhibits healthy living
3 Expansion of school/wider community links.

In terms of evaluating the success of health promotion and education in schools, Lister-Sharpe et al. (1999) carried out a systematic review, and concluded that school health promotion and education programmes can have a significant impact on children's health and behaviour, although they do not do so consistently. They noted that most interventions were able to increase health-related knowledge and change behavioural intentions, but that changes in attitudes and health behaviours are harder to achieve. In terms of smoking, for example, health promotion in schools has led to a reduction in intention to smoke and to some postponement of initiation of smoking, but has rarely influenced long-term smoking rates.

Health promotion in the workplace

For those in employment, work is a key part of life. Knobel (1983), for instance, estimated that it is possible to reach 85 per cent of the US population via the worksite, and similar proportions must apply in other countries in the western world. It is not surprising, therefore, that delivering health education to the workforce is a key aspect of governments' health promotion strategies. As the UK's Department of Health (1999) noted in their White Paper, the environment in which we work influences our health choices and can be a force for improving health – for individuals and the communities of which they are part. As part of setting its priorities for improving public health, the Department of Health emphasized a commitment to improving the working conditions to reduce the causes of ill health related to work, and to promoting the work environment as a source of better health.

The UK White Paper followed the establishment of the European Network for Workplace Health Promotion (Federal Institute for Occupational Safety and Health, 1996). The network identified five key priorities for action:

1 Increased awareness of workplace health promotion, and the promotion of responsibility for health with regard to all stakeholders
2 Identification and dissemination of models of good practice
3 Development of guidelines for effective workplace health promotion
4 Ensuring commitment of members states to incorporate principles of workplace health promotion in their respective policies
5 Addressing the specific challenges of working effectively with small and medium-sized enterprises (see Tones and Tilford, 2001).

Similar commitments and efforts have been made in the USA and many Australasian countries.

Systematic reviews have shown that the introduction of health education and promotion into the workplace has led to many successes but, as with schools, the effects have been inconsistent (e.g. Peersman et al., 1998). The most successful initiatives have been the introduction of risk-assessment and screening programmes, with a choice of education programmes, whereas the least effective have been weight-control programmes. In general, interventions have been found to be more successful when they were associated with individualized delivery of information.

Health education and communication

Whether it occurs in schools, the workplace or elsewhere, health promotion is the product of health education and health public policy (Tones, 1998). Health education is any intentional activity which is designed to achieve health- or illness-related learning, that is, some relatively permanent change in an individual's capability or disposition. Effective health education can have many significant (positive) effects. Thus, it can produce changes in knowledge and understanding or ways of thinking; it can influence or clarify values; it can bring about some shifts in beliefs or attitudes; it can facilitate the learning of new skills; and, importantly, it can lead to desired changes in behaviour or lifestyle (Tones and Tilford, 2001).

Clearly, effective communication is key to effective health education. There are numerous ways in which this communication can occur. Some of the most common are via written Patient Information Leaflets, product labelling, the Internet, and media campaigns. Before looking at each of these in more detail, we will consider three general strategies or approaches to health promotion that can be taken.

Health promotion strategies

Most countries have focused their efforts on primary prevention activities through the modification of lifestyle factors that account for the greatest share of the burden of disease (e.g. smoking, excess alcohol, poor diet and risky sexual behaviour). Key methods that have been used to address these include health education, fiscal and legislative measures (such as increased tax on cigarettes and alcohol, and compulsory wearing of car seatbelts) and environmental changes (such as the introduction of airbags into cars, and the removal of asbestos from old buildings). Interestingly, comparisons of the effectiveness of public health strategies that have used education/persuasion with those that have used financial or legal changes have shown the latter to be far more effective (e.g. Stroebe, 2000). Clearly, however, it is difficult to apply financial and legal sanctions to many aspects of unhealthy living.

Marks et al. (2000) outlined three main strategies or approaches to health promotion. These are the Behavioural Change approach, the Self-empowerment approach, and the Collective Action approach.

The Behavioural Change approach

The key objective of this approach is to bring about changes in the behaviour of individuals through changing their cognitions (thoughts and beliefs). This typically requires increasing people's knowledge about the causes of health and illness through the provision of information about health risks and hazards. The Behavioural Change approach is based on the assumption that people are rational decision makers and that their health behaviours are informed by their cognitions. Thus, applying social cognition models, such as the Health Belief Model (e.g. Rosenstock, 1974; see Chapter 3), to plan health interventions would be an example of this approach to health promotion. Limitations of this approach include its focus on the cognitions of individuals, its failure to take sufficient account of individual differences, and the fact that it has not had much success in targeting important socio-economic causes of ill health.

The Self-empowerment approach

The main objective of this approach is to empower people to make healthy choices so that they can increase control over their physical, social and internal environments. This is mostly done through participatory learning techniques (such as group work, counselling and social skills training). It is based on the assumption that power is a universal resource that can be used by everyone. However, a limitation is that it seems to ignore the fact that there are systematic inequalities that are known to exist with regard to access to material and psychological resources. Like the previous approach, the Self-empowerment approach has also been criticized for focusing on the individual as 'the target for change'.

The Collective Action approach

The main aim of this third approach to health promotion is to improve public health by addressing the important socio-economic and environmental determinants of health. Specifically, the key objective is to modify the relevant social, economic and physical structures that generate ill health. In order to achieve this, however, individuals must act collectively to improve their social and physical environments. The Collective Action approach is therefore based on the assumption that individuals share sufficient interests to allow them to act in the necessary collective way. As should be apparent, this third approach is more 'political' than the other two approaches and, to be effective, can require significant resources.

Clearly, effective communication is central to all three approaches. However, the particular way in which it is applied will differ according to which approach is taken. Thus, the content of the message, and the way in which it is presented, will differ according to whether the main aim of the activity is to change individual behaviour, empower people or to address major socio-economic and environmental determinants of health. An important point to note is that communication in all cases involves more that simply getting a message across. Rather, it involves building relationships and empowering people so that they can make appropriate health-related choices and decisions (Katz et al., 2000).

Patient Information Leaflets

Despite the considerable growth in the availability of computerized health information systems and access to health information via the Internet, written Patient Information Leaflets (PILs) are still one of the most common forms of disseminating information about illnesses and treatments. The Arthritis and Rheumatism Council in the UK, for example, produce over 1.5 million leaflets per year. This growth in the availability of PILs is due to several factors, including increased regulation (such as in relation to medicines), increased activities by self-help and other support groups, and enhanced public awareness and expectations (see also Mossman et al., 1999). Patient Information Leaflets serve a number of purposes (Coulter et al., 1998). These include promoting better health and preventing disease, encouraging self-care and reducing inappropriate service use, ensuring the appropriateness of treatment decisions and improving the effectiveness of clinical care.

The effects of providing written information

Several researchers have argued that providing information in written form is more effective than via spoken communications (e.g. Ley, 1988; Ley and Llewellyn, 1995; Raynor, 1998). What are now considered to be classic studies of Ley (1973), for example, showed that after five minutes, patients forgot about half of the spoken information given to them in the consultation. Similarly, Wilson et al. (1992) found that, after 24 hours, patients could remember only a third of the spoken information given to them by pharmacists. However, there is also evidence that the combination of the two forms of information can be more effective than providing written information alone. Johnson and Sandford (2004), for instance, found that providing a combination of written and spoken health information for patients being discharged from acute hospital settings was more effective in improving patient knowledge and satisfaction, than was providing spoken information alone. Raynor (1998) suggested that the combination of the two forms of information can maximize effectiveness through mechanisms such as repetition, reinforcement and signalling importance. In addition, Morris (1989) argued that the strongest beneficial effects are often when written information is combined with other educational interventions, such as videos, talks and one-to-one spoken communications. This argument was supported by Semple and McGowan (2002) when they suggested that, in many situations, written information should be used to supplement and reinforce information obtained from direct contact with health professionals.

Whether used in isolation, or in combination with other methods, it is generally acknowledged that a major benefit of written leaflets is that they can be referred to by patients (or by their relatives) when they are away from the stressful environment of the consultation room. This allows patients to 'refresh and review their knowledge at all stages of their condition' (Kenny et al., 1998, p. 473). Raynor (1998, p. 86) suggested that written information has the potential to influence health behaviours in at least three different ways, in that it can influence:

♦ patients who want to follow the recommended treatment but need more information to do so
♦ patients who have fears and misconceptions that need countering
♦ patients who are dissatisfied with their care.

Thus, written information materials can be aimed at providing specific instructions, influencing beliefs, and/or generally increasing satisfaction. A number of studies have shown that many leaflets do have positive effects on patients' knowledge and health outcomes. Bishop et al. (1996), for instance, found that people with rheumatoid arthritis who received a written information leaflet showed an increase in knowledge about their condition, and reported less pain and decreased depression. A follow-on study showed that the short-term increase in knowledge was maintained over a six-month period (Barlow and Wright, 1998). Benefits were also reported by Mac-Farlane et al. (1997), who found that issuing a written leaflet to patients with respiratory infections reduced their reconsultation rates. Similarly, a more recent study by Coudeyre et al. (2002) found that the provision of leaflets for low back pain patients undergoing steroid injections under fluoroscopy reduced state anxiety and increased patients' knowledge and satisfaction with the information provided.

Not all studies have reported such beneficial effects, however. Turner and Williams (2002), for example, reported that older adults who were given a written leaflet, following the provision of spoken information during a consultation, had forgotten most of it after six weeks. Similarly, Brown et al. (2003) found that recall of surgical complications from otologic surgery was equally poor both with written and spoken information, and that the poor performance was independent of age and education.

Assessment of existing Patient Information Leaflets

Despite the positive results reported earlier, it must be recognized that the provision of written information is not likely to have a positive effect on health behaviours and outcomes if it is of poor quality or not easily accessible. Detrimental effects can occur if people are given unclear, conflicting, overly complex or too much information. In 1993 a survey by the Audit Commission in the UK found several inadequacies in the quality and availability of written information for patients. The Commission made a number of recommendations for improving the situation, specifically suggesting that clinical staff and general managers should work together to:

◆ review the written information currently distributed, as well as the distribution mechanisms
◆ find out what kind of information patients and relatives want to be given
◆ provide written information about conditions, procedures and post-operative care
◆ make written information from national organizations available to patients and caregivers
◆ allocate resources to help fund the production and purchase of written information
◆ make clear arrangements for distributing written information at the right time.

To be effective, a leaflet must be noticed, read, understood, believed and remembered (Kenny et al., 1998). Unfortunately a national survey of written information given to patients in the UK (Payne et al., 2000) showed that 64 per cent of leaflets could be understood by only 40 per cent of the population. In addition, many of the leaflets did not meet basic guidelines for legibility and readability. Coulter et al. (1998, p. 16) listed a number of criteria that have been recommended for evaluating the quality of PILs, including:

♦ accessibility
♦ acceptability
♦ readability and comprehensibility
♦ style and attractiveness of presentation
♦ accuracy and reliability of content
♦ coverage and comprehensiveness
♦ currency and arrangements for editorial review
♦ references to sources and strength of evidence
♦ where to find further information
♦ credibility of authors, publishers, sponsors
♦ relevance and utility.

Coulter et al (1998) reported a large-scale study which assessed the extent and nature of information materials available for patients for 10 common health problems (for example, back pain, depression, infertility), as well as assessing the quality of the materials. Initial focus group discussions identified a number of different purposes for which patients reported needing good-quality PILs. These included: the need to understand what is wrong with them, to gain a realistic picture of their likely prognosis and to understand the processes and likely outcomes of potential tests and treatments. In addition, the information should aid people in self-care, inform them about available services and sources of support, and help them to identify the best healthcare providers. Finally, they wanted PILs to provide reassurance and to help other people to understand their condition and its treatment.

Overall, the study's findings gave cause for concern in relation to both the availability and quality of existing PILs. In particular, it was found that most patients did not receive the information about treatment options that they needed to participate in decision making. In addition, the quality of most of the reviewed patient information materials was unsatisfactory. Specifically, many contained inaccurate and outdated information and few provided appropriate information about treatment risks and side effects. Topics of relevance were often not included and coverage of treatment options was incomplete. Furthermore, technical terms were not explained, uncertainties were either glossed over or ignored, and information about the effectiveness of different treatments was often unreliable or missing. Finally, it was noted that few of the materials actively promoted shared decision making (Coulter et al., 1998). Similar findings to this were reported by Meredith et al. (1995) who examined 25 leaflets, and contrasted the information given with the information wanted by 5361 patients. They reported that much of the information had considerable shortcomings. Specifically, it lacked uniformity in form and content, topics of relevance to patients were limited, terminology was often poor and the patients' experiences were often at variance with what their doctors had told them.

More recently, Brown et al. (2004) carried out a study in 12 ophthalmology departments in the West Midlands, UK, to assess the extent to which the provision of PILs before cataract surgery provide patients with enough information to give adequately informed consent. The leaflets were scored according to the information that they provided on diagnosis, prognosis, treatment options, costs to patient, details about the procedure, its purpose, likely benefits, how to prepare for it, what to expect during and after the operation, and common as well as serious complications that might occur. Readability was also assessed. Brown et al found that all the leaflets provided information on diagnosis, lifestyle changes required post-operatively and cost to patient. However, only five units had leaflets that mentioned the risks involved in cataract surgery. The other areas of information were covered in between 50 and 75 per cent of leaflets. The average readability score of the leaflets was also high. In line with this, White et al. (2004) found that nearly half of the leaflets about hayfever that were available in GP surgeries and community pharmacies in South-East England, did not show the date of publication, and one-third of those that did were more than five years old. Fewer than half contained information on the full range of management and treatment options, and all had readability scores requiring at least secondary school education. In addition, the researchers found that no leaflets at all were available in 30 per cent of the community pharmacies and 23 per cent of the GP practices they surveyed.

On the basis of their study's findings, Coulter et al. (1998, p. xi) made the following recommendations in relation to producing PILs:

♦ involve patients throughout the development process
♦ involve a wide range of clinical experts
♦ be specific about the purpose of information and the target audience
♦ consider information needs of minority groups
♦ review clinical research evidence and use systematic review
♦ plan how materials can support shared decision making
♦ consider cost and feasibility when selecting media
♦ develop a strategy for distribution
♦ evaluate materials and how they are used
♦ publicise availability.

In terms of the actual content of the materials, they recommended that, developers should:

♦ use patient questions as a starting point
♦ ensure that common concerns and misconceptions are addressed

- refer to all relevant treatment or management options
- include honest information about risks and benefits
- include quantitative information where possible
- include checklists and questions to ask the doctor, and sources of further information
- use non-alarmist, non-patronising language in an active voice
- use structured and concise text with good illustrations
- include references and publication date.

(p. xi)

Many of Coulter et al's recommendations are in line with those of a number of other researchers and practitioners (e.g. Kitching, 1990; Newton et al., 1998; Raynor, 1998; Wright, 1998). In general, there is a consensus of opinion that the extent to which prose is comprehended is determined largely by the complexity of the sentences and the familiarity of the vocabulary. Thus, when producing written information materials, technical terms should be replaced by everyday counterparts, non-essential information should be eliminated, word and sentence length should be reduced, language structures should be simplified and information reordered to enhance coherence. Kenny et al. (1998) recommended that all new Patient Information Leaflets should declare an objective score of readability using a standard formula. In relation to this, Albert and Chadwick (1992) suggested that leaflets should not exceed a readability age of 12. However, in aiming for simplicity, authors have to be careful that leaflets do not end up becoming overly patronizing.

In addition, as Newton et al. (1998) pointed out, to be meaningful, the leaflet content must relate to the reader's existing knowledge. One way of doing this is to use appropriate analogies and concrete examples. In terms of design and layout, materials should incorporate clear headings and use of bullet points, plenty of white space, and the font should be clear and at least 12 point size. Finally, in order to be believed, the clinical content of a leaflet should be correct, balanced, unbiased and developed independently of commercial interests. Overall, there is now clear advice from a variety of sources on 'how to write a good leaflet' with respect to style, language, layout, print size, readability, diagrams, colour and numeracy. This includes a number of articles and publications that review the evidence for this advice (e.g. Centre for Health Quality Improvement, 1997; Kenny et al., 1998; Newton et al., 1998).

As a general principle, Wright (1998) has suggested that information design needs to be reader based rather than text based (see also Schriver, 1997). Wright emphasized that it is essential to carry out a thorough evaluation of any materials that are produced, and that the process must be intimately involved with the development of the materials (rather than a separate process that is tagged on at the end). In a similar vein, Mayberry and Mayberry (1996) proposed that the scientific evaluation of patient information must include tests of both readability and comprehension, as well as of the long-term effects of the material. Wright (1998) argued that evaluation requires more than just showing the material to a few people and asking them if they like it or find it helpful. One reason is that people may 'like' leaflets that do not actually lead to good understanding or retention. A study by Livingstone et al. (1993), for instance, found that 90 per cent of 312 people evaluating a leaflet about cystic fibrosis said that they found it easy to understand but, nevertheless, more than one-third gave the wrong answer when asked about the likelihood that they might have the cystic fibrosis gene. Thus, Wright (1998) recommended that performance-based criteria are needed when evaluating materials. In terms of medicine information leaflets, for example, some specific criteria could be that a certain percentage of people (e.g. 70 per cent) can locate relevant dosage information within a specified time (e.g. 20 seconds), that 80 per cent of readers can demonstrate correct understanding for responding to a hypothetical scenario, and that, say, 90 per cent of readers can identify the circumstances in which the medicine should be taken. More broadly, Sless (2001) has noted that setting performance benchmarks for written information for patients involves establishing technical, social, physical, aesthetic and usability criteria. Clearly, therefore, such evaluations need to be well planned and rigorously carried out.

Medicine information leaflets

Written patient information is probably most associated with the distribution of medicines. Medicine information leaflets (often referred to as Patient Package Inserts in Europe) are now routinely provided with the majority of prescribed and over-the-counter medicines in many countries in the western world. In the USA, the growing availability of medicine information leaflets followed a Federal mandate which stated that by the year 2000 useful information must be delivered to 75 per cent of patients receiving new prescriptions. The intention was that this would rise to 95 per cent by 2006 (US Department of Health and Human Services, 1996). The Federal Drug Administration (FDA) steering committee recommended that all information provided to the public must be scientifically accurate, unbiased, easily understood and comprehensive enough to be useful to patients (Marwick, 1997). The preferred route for delivering the information in the USA has been through computer-generated leaflets from community pharmacies. Unfortunately, a survey commissioned by the FDA (Traynor, 2002) found that, although 89 per cent of newly filled prescriptions came with written information for consumers, much of the information was incomplete and of limited use to patients. Using predetermined criteria, a panel of 16 pharmacy professionals found that 51 per cent or fewer of the leaflets provided adequate information about contra-indications to the prescribed drug. In addition, no more than 53 per cent of the leaflets provided sufficient warning of adverse events, and 45 per cent or fewer described important precautions patients should take when using drugs.

Following this, the FDA (2006) have recently revised their guidelines for prescription drug information. In addition to improved graphical specifications, the new format requires the insertion of a new highlights section that gives immediate access to the most important information about medicine risks and benefits, a table of contents and the date of initial product approval. The aim is to give patients and healthcare professionals clear and concise prescription information in order to manage the risks of medicine use and reduce medical errors.

Likewise, in Australia, legislation was introduced in 1993 which required all new medicines to be accompanied by information leaflets (referred to as 'consumer medicines information'). Information in the leaflet has to be consistent with the information in the drug's Data Sheet, although not all of the information in the Data Sheet has to be included in the leaflet. As in the USA, the preferred route for delivery of the medicines information has been through computer-generated leaflets in community pharmacies (Raynor, 2001). In order to exert control over the quality of leaflets, guidelines were commissioned for writing and testing leaflets (Dowling, 1996; Sless, 2001). The guidelines specify, for example, that any literate patient should be able to find at least 90 per cent of what he or she is looking for in the leaflet and should be able to understand 90 per cent of what they find. Sless (2001) noted that the guidelines had been used to develop over 800 consumer medicines information leaflets to date, covering most major therapeutic classes of prescription medicine.

In some European countries, medicines information leaflets have been available for some time. This is particularly the case in The Netherlands, Sweden, France and Germany, although the content and method of distribution varies. The general tradition, however, has been to incorporate leaflets as package inserts, rather than to generate them on line in community pharmacies. In many cases, the content of the leaflets is fairly technical (Dickinson et al. 2001). In an attempt to increase the availability of materials, and to ensure a degree of consistency, the European Commission issued a Directive in 1992 (European Commission, 1992), which required that all medicines supplied to patients should be accompanied by a comprehensive information leaflet which must include a list of all side effects referred to in the medicine's Summary of Product Characteristics (previously known as Data Sheet), in a form that is understandable to the patient. The Directive came fully into effect in Europe in 1999, following a phasing-in period. It was implemented in the UK through the development of a patient pack dispensing system (that is, the incorporation of patient package inserts).

In 1996 the European Commission (EC) produced a *Draft Guideline* on assessing readability (together with a model leaflet) to be used by manufacturers when producing leaflets. The recommended method was based on that used in Australia (Sless and Wiseman, 1994) and involved interviews with potential users to ascertain whether they could find specified key information in the leaflet quickly and easily, and whether they could understand and act upon it. It was recommended that the leaflet would be deemed to be satisfactory if more than 80 per cent of consumers could use it successfully according to these two criteria.

Dickinson et al. (2001) carried out an empirical study to evaluate the EC's proposals for producing PILs. They compared people's ability to use two specially constructed leaflets that were based on either the EC model leaflet or on recognized best practice in information design. Their test involved requiring participants to find and understand 15 key pieces of information in each leaflet (e.g. when the medicine should be taken, how it should be stored and what to do if too much is taken). The results showed that performance was worse with the EC model leaflet; the criterion that 80 per cent of readers should be able to locate and understand the requested information was only reached for 3 of the 15 items, compared with 8 for the leaflet that was based on best practice in information design. Subsequent interviews with the participants confirmed many of the difficulties with the EC leaflet, including the fact that many of readers did not understand the information that they were given about drug interactions and contra-indications for use.

In order to assess the extent to which leaflets were being used by con-sumers following implementation of the Directive, Raynor and Knapp (2000) carried out a study in community pharmacies in Leeds (UK). Patients were recruited as they collected their prescriptions and were telephoned seven days later for a structured interview. The interviews showed that leaflets were not provided with one-third of the prescriptions that were collected. Of those that were provided, 17 per cent of the sample reported that they had taken no notice of the leaflet, and 26 per cent said that they had not kept it. Only 40 per cent of the sample said that they had read some of the leaflet, and only 20 per cent said that they had read all of it. Finally, only 7 patients out of the sample of 215 reported taking an action as a direct result of reading the leaflet (e.g. returning to the pharmacy or GP). More recently, Hughes et al. (2002) found that, although the majority of partici-pants in their study had received a medicine information leaflet when pur-chasing an over-the-counter medicine, only a small number had actually read it. The most common reason given for not reading it was that it was not the first time that they had purchased the medicine. People were more likely to have read the leaflet if the medicine was new to them, or if they had experienced a particular adverse effect.

In 1998, the European Commission published a further *Guideline* (European Commission, 1998) to standardize the way in which information about the frequency of occurrence of medication side effects is described in PILs. The Guideline recommended that the frequency of side effects could be banded into five groupings, based on five verbal descriptors, ranging from 'very rare' to 'very common', with each term being associated with a specified range of frequencies of occurrence, as shown in Figure 7.1. Thus, according to the Guideline, a side effect should be described as being 'common', for example, if it occurs in between 1 and 10 per cent of people who take the medicine.

Unfortunately, the EC's recommendations were not based on sound empirical evidence, nor were they evaluated prior to implementation. As mentioned in the previous chapter, a series of studies by my research group showed that members of the general public, patients and doctors consistently overestimated the likelihood of side effects occurring when the probabilities were described using the EC recommended descriptors. For example, although the EC recommended that a side effect should be considered to be 'common' if it occurred in 'between 1 and 10 per cent of people who take the medicine', our studies showed that people estimate the level of risk of 'common' side effects to be around 50 per cent (e.g. Berry et al., 2002, 2003, 2004; Knapp et al., 2004).

More recently, the EC has updated its regulations (European Commission, 2005) in relation to the preparation of PILs. The modifications are relatively minor, mostly focusing on changes to the order of information in the PIL, and the additional need for systematic user testing before leaflets are published and distributed.

As noted earlier, it is important not to give patients either too little or too much information on PILs. Clearly, what would be considered to be the 'right' amount of information will depend on a number of factors, including the educational level of the recipients and the health behaviour in question.

Verbal descriptor	EU assigned frequency
Very common	> 10%
Common	1–10%
Uncommon	0.1–1%
Rare	0.01–0.1%
Very rare	< 0.01%

Figure 7.1 EU-recommended verbal descriptors together with assigned probability ranges

As far as medicines are concerned, the International Medicine Benefit/Risk Foundation (IMBRF, 1993) recommended that the minimum information patients should be given should cover the medicine's name and dose, its purpose and benefit, how it should be taken, and special precautions and adverse effects. Similarly, Mottram and Reed (1997) pointed out that patients need to know certain points of information in order to avoid harm and to derive full benefit from their prescriptions. This information includes how to take the drug, how to store it, how it is expected to help, how to recognize problems, such as adverse effects, and what to do about them if they occur.

In addition to disseminating health information via PILs, important information also needs to be conveyed on product labels. This not only applies to medicines but also to the foods that we eat. Research is increasingly showing clear links between inadequacies in diet and health problems.

Nutritional labelling and health claims on food products

Many food products now feature labels that convey important nutritional and health-related information. In recent years there has been an increased emphasis on the use and regulation of such product labelling. The UK government's recent White Paper on public health, for example, expressed a commitment to working with the food industry to develop better information on nutritional content on packaged food. This included the intention to introduce a clear coding system that would be in common use by 2006, and that busy people could understand at a glance (Department of Health, 2004). Improvements have also been brought about through increased controls on communication, such as restrictions on product advertising. Again the UK White Paper has committed to restricted advertising and promotion to children of food and drinks that are high in fat, salt and sugar, as well as further restrictions on advertising of tobacco, including banning advertising on the Internet, and reducing the size of tobacco advertisements that are allowed in shops.

Nutritional and health claims on foods clearly have the potential to contribute to the achievement of public health objectives. Basically, a nutritional claim means 'any representation that states, suggests, or implies that a food has particular nutritional properties including, but not limited to, the energy value and content of the protein, fat and carbohydrates, as well as the content of vitamins and minerals' (Richardson et al., 2003, p. 100). In contrast, a health claim means 'any representation that states, suggests, or implies that a relationship exists between a food, or constituent of that food, and health' (p. 100). Richardson (2005) proposes that nutrition and health claims can exert an effect on consumer behaviour to an extent that consumers:

◆ are aware of the claim
◆ understand the claim

- make appropriate health inferences from the claim
- consider the claim credible
- attach attitudinal relevance to the claim, that is, the claims are appealing and motivating
- translate the claim into action, for example purchase intent.

Many countries in the western world now regulate the information that appears on nutritional labels and in health claims. Generally, there is more consensus over the former, whereas health claims are far more controversial. Within the European Union, the use of health claims on products is only allowed if there has been a thorough scientific evaluation of the evidence for the claim.

Clearly, food labels of either sort will only be beneficial if they are presented in a format that consumers can readily understand. In line with this, Richardson et al. (2003) suggested that health claims must not only be truthful, but that they should be unambiguous and understandable for the intended consumer. In addition, they must make clear that the claim applies only to food consumed in the context of a total dietary pattern and should not encourage over-consumption of a given food. Probably not surprisingly, empirical evidence suggests that consumers often have difficulty understanding many food labels. An additional problem for public health is that they are predominantly read and 'used' by a relatively limited sector of the population, such as younger adults, women, more highly educated people and those with a particular interest in health and nutrition. At present, therefore, the effectiveness of nutritional labelling tends to rely largely on a motivated and educated public to make healthy choices. Clearly, if nutritional labels are to be a more widespread public health tool, more needs to be done to ensure their applicability to a larger proportion of the population.

Disseminating health information via the media

The mass media play an important role in disseminating health information to the general public in much of the western world. Nowadays, the media enable information on a whole range of health topics to be conveyed straight into the homes of a large proportion of the population. This may be done via news reports in the written press and on radio and television (such as when a new health scare breaks out), feature articles in magazines and newspapers, radio and television documentaries, and the increasing number of television soap operas and 'docu-soaps'. The latter often take the form of the televization of a typical day, or week, in an accident and emergency department, for example, or on a hospital's children's ward.

Two distinct models of health education via the mass media were identified by Redman et al. (1990). These are the 'direct effect' model and the 'agenda setting' model. In the case of the former, the objective is to change or prevent harmful behaviour and promote positive health behaviours, using similar types of direct method as might be used by an individual health professional. In contrast, in the 'agenda setting' model, the media are used to raise awareness of a health problem or to gain support for a particular health-related public policy. Some health campaigns, such as drink drive campaigns, often use a mixture of both methods.

Clearly, the growing influence of the media can be considered to be positive or negative, depending on the particular circumstances (and irrespective of whichever of the above two models is used). On the positive side, the media can be very good at raising awareness of particular health issues, and for reducing the amount of stigma associated with some illnesses. Richard Nixon, former US President, once remarked that 'American people don't believe anything until they see it on TV' (Chrystal, 2005, p. 155), and there may be some truth in this (and not just in the USA). Many fictional television programmes that feature a particular health issue (such as cancer, therapeutic abortion and AIDs/HIV) often include an information or help-line number at the end of the programme. A number of studies have shown that the organizations concerned often report a record number of calls immediately after such shows have been broadcast. Marcus (2000), for example, reported that after an episode of the US television programme, *General Hospital*, the National Cancer Institute confirmed that 207 callers responded to the public service announcement that followed the programme.

Unfortunately, the media can have less positive influences. Many popular characters in fictional programmes, such as television soap operas, often portray negative role models as far as health behaviours are concerned. Signorelli (1993), for instance, noted that characters on popular television shows consistently role model unhealthy behaviours, such as overeating high-calorie, high-sodium and high-fat foods, snacking and eating on the move. Similarly, analysis showed that characters drank alcohol more than twice as often as tea or coffee and 15 times more often than water.

As far as news items are concerned, the media still often disseminate incomplete, biased or inaccurate information. Although we can all have some sympathy with Dame Rose Macaulay's suggestion that 'you should always believe all you read in newspapers as this makes them more interesting' (Chrystal, 2005, p. 137), one does need to be cautious. Moynihan et al. (2000), for example, analysed 207 US news media stories (relating to three different drugs) that appeared between 1994 and 1998, and found that the majority included inadequate or incomplete information about the risks, benefits and costs of the medicines. Similarly, Carlson et al. (1997) found that more than two-thirds of reports of the study of breast cancer and mammography contained factual inaccuracies.

One point noted by Moynihan et al. (2000) was that over 80 per cent of the articles only reported information about risks and benefits of the medicines in 'relative' terms. However, referring to the 'doubled risk of cancer', for example, without indicating what the actual size of the risk is, can be very misleading. Indeed, as we saw in the previous chapter, the 1995 'pill scare' in the UK was greatly exacerbated by the media, who emphasized the doubled risk of thrombosis that was associated with taking the third-generation oral contraceptive, without mentioning that the absolute level of risk was still extremely low. Such biased reporting was also apparent in reports of the more recent hormone replacement therapy scare (Paling, 2004).

In defence of the media, Bennett (1998) pointed out that the media do not usually create public interest. Rather, they simply amplify (albeit sometimes to a considerable degree) existing public interest in particular 'forms of mishap'. Thus, the public and the media reinforce each other in a negative way. Bennett (1998) identified a number of 'media triggers' that he suggested determine the extent of coverage that is given to a particular issue. These include questions of blame, alleged secrets or cover-ups, human interest, links with high-profile issues or personalities and the existence of conflict. In addition, media interest is greater when a large number of people are, or could be, affected by the health risk in question.

Communication via computers and the Internet

People in the developed world are increasingly using computers to communicate information. This increased usage is recognized to have advantages and disadvantages. Computers allow interactions to take place over large distances and across time zones, and with a large number of people. However, computer-mediated communication can suppress the amount of information that is exchanged, which in turn can lead to poorer communication outcomes (e.g. Hollingshead, 1996). Similarly, by restricting paralanguage and non-verbal communication, it can detrimentally affect interactions, particularly between participants who have a closer relationship (Hollingshead, 1998). In general, however, people do adapt to the mode of communication with time, and often respond as it if were not computer mediated (e.g. Walther, 1996).

Computers are being increasingly used in health communication. Health professionals now frequently communicate with each other via e-mail. Computers can also be used to aid decision making by both health professionals and patients (see, for example, O'Connor and Edwards, 2001; O'Connor et al., 2003), and for patient-education purposes, complementing more traditional spoken and leaflet-based approaches. Many public places, such as supermarkets, community centres and medical practices, house computers running health-related programmes. Although few would argue that computers are an effective replacement for personal contact between healthcare providers and patients, there is evidence that they can play a useful complementary role. As Bental et al. (1999), noted, many patients find information access using a computer acceptable and, sometimes, less embarrassing than having to interact directly with healthcare providers.

One advantage of computers, compared with written communications, is that they can be used interactively. Thus, consumers using a computer health information system can input personal data and receive timely and appropriate responses and advice. Many studies in the field of education have shown that people are generally more motivated and learn better in interactive settings. A second advantage of computers is that they can be used to provide information that is tailored, or personalized, to a particular individual. Whereas the majority of written health information (e.g. Patient Information Leaflets, campaign posters) is generic, computers can be used to provide information that has taken account of the particular patient's background, knowledge, needs and preferences.

Tailored systems have now been developed in several medical domains, including asthma, diabetes, migraine, cancer and dental treatments. A number of studies have shown that use of tailored systems is beneficial as tailored communications are generally better remembered than generic ones and are more effective for influencing behaviour change (e.g. Kreuter and Holt, 2001; Skinner et al., 1999; Straus, 2002). Kreuter et al. (1999) argued that there is a strong public health rationale for tailoring materials, and that computer-tailored health communications should be viewed as a tool of public health communicators to be incorporated into comprehensive programmes of health promotion, disease prevention and disease management.

Although computers offer these potential benefits in the field of health communication, it has to be recognized that not everyone can gain easy access to computerized health information (e.g. Fogel, 2003). Even in the twenty-first century, there still exists a 'digital divide' between those who have access and those who do not. Moreover, many of the latter (such as the elderly and those from lower socio-economic classes) often have the most need of healthcare and health-related information. This is referred to as the 'inverse information law' (Eysenbach, 2000), in that access to appropriate information is particularly difficult for those who need it most.

The Internet

The most common use of computers today in relation to health communication is to gain access to the Internet. Over the past 20 years, the Internet has become a global communication network that is now accessed by tens of millions of users. The Office of National Statistics in the UK, for example, reported that, in spring 2004, 11.7 million households in Britain (that is, 47 per cent of all households) had access to the Internet (ONS, 2004), and this number is likely to have increased since then. Through the Internet, increasing numbers of the general population and healthcare professionals can gain free and easy access to vast amounts of health-related information that was previously unavailable. It has been noted by Levy and Strombeck (2002), for example, that 'health and medicine' is the fourth most popular 'on-line subject' and that there are well over 20 000 different Internet sites that provide health-related information. A survey of over 500 patients enrolled in a primary care practice in the USA (Diaz et al., 2002) showed that over 50 per cent of respondents regularly used the Internet to obtain medical information. Similarly, Fox and Fallows (2003) reported that over 80 per cent of adult Internet users have accessed the Internet for general health information, with 36 per cent seeking information about medicines. If anything, this level of usage is likely to have increased since then.

Research has shown that sufferers of a serious illness, such as cancer, are particularly inclined to access information about their disease via the Internet (e.g. Whitte et al., 2005). A recent qualitative study of 175 adult cancer patients found that the patients used the Internet for a wide range of informational and support needs through all stages of cancer care, from diagnosis to follow-up treatment (Ziebland et al., 2004). The patients liked the privacy of the Internet, as well as the ability to obtain reassurance that their doctor was doing the right thing for them. Many also felt that it helped them to display competence and social fitness in the face of their illness.

Not surprisingly, this massive increase in access to health-related information can have advantages and disadvantages for health communication. On the positive side, it can enable health professionals to gain easy access to up-to-date research findings about illnesses and potential treatments. It can also lead to increased patient knowledge, which may result in early detection of particular conditions and improved self-care and treatment management, as well as access to relevant support groups and organizations. As noted by Jadad (1999), the Internet should have a significant effect on the way doctors and patients interact, in that it 'will foster a new level of knowledge among patients, enable them to have input into making decisions about their healthcare, and allow them to participate in active partnerships with various groups of decision makers' (p. 761). Thus, the Internet can function as a great leveller by placing lay persons on virtually equal footing with scientific and technical experts (Horsch and Harding, 1997).

On the negative side, however, this increased access to information can lead to increased confusion and anxiety in users, particularly when conflicting information and advice is available (or when information that they have found themselves conflicts with advice from their healthcare provider). Petrie and Wessely (2002) argued that the Internet has led to the spread of information about health scares and has brought a new dimension to patients' worries in relation to these. Furthermore, not all healthcare professionals (particularly doctors) are happy with their patients accessing additional sources of information and being more proactive in their healthcare. As Hardey (1999) observed, the Internet can represent a challenge to the previously hierarchical model of information giving, with a shift in control and a decline in awe of doctors by patients. Many doctors do not like (and can feel upstaged or threatened by) being faced with patients who bring information downloaded from the Internet to their consultations (Jadad, 1999).

One of the biggest problems with using the Internet to access health-related information is that there is no guarantee that the information is accurate or reliable. Indeed, Berland et al. (2001) reviewed a large number of US health information sites and found that many offered incomplete, misleading or difficult-to-understand information, or blurred the distinction between providing information and advice and companies advertising their own products. Clearly, widespread access to inaccurate and misleading information can pose a public health threat. In this context, Eng (2001) suggested that some of the consequences of poor quality Internet information include 'inappropriate treatment or delays in seeking appropriate healthcare and damage to the patient provider relationship' (p. 12). One reason for the wide variation in quality of information available is that currently anyone can post health-related information on the Internet, regardless of their personal expertise or intentions (Levy and Strombeck, 2002). Although some commercial organizations have produced codes of practice for helping to ensure information quality and reliability, there is currently no obligation for information providers to use these.

Clearly, an issue for healthcare providers is that they frequently have no idea about what other information sources their patients have accessed and the level of (both accurate and inaccurate) knowledge they possess. Furthermore, the time-limited nature of most consultations often means that healthcare providers interact with the patient without being able to take account of this and adapt their communications accordingly. On occasion, this can lead to patients feeling frustrated and confused.

Designing effective health messages

Whether information is distributed in written form or via the media and/or the Internet, the message needs to be effectively designed. Some simple guidelines in relation to the graphical presentation of written forms of dissemination were presented earlier. More generally, as noted by Maibach and Parrott (1995), an essential first step is to get people to attend to the message. Louis and Sutton (1991) found that people are more likely to engage actively in message processing if the content is unusual or unfamiliar, if it represents a discrepancy between expectations and reality, and when an external or internal request causes an individual to initiate an increased level of conscious attention. Thus Maibach and Parrott (1995) recommended that communicators should use novel messages, settings and media to present health messages, and that they should consider the use of discrepant and unexpected messages, media and settings. In addition, they should instruct the audience to pay attention to the message.

Hale and Dillard (1995) suggested that the use of fear appeals is often a successful method of disseminating health information to the wider public. Fear appeals are persuasive messages that emphasize the harmful physical or social consequences of failing to comply with the message's recommendations. Hale and Dillard argued that fear appeals have enormous persuasive potential and can promote better health. They suggested that, to be effective, a fear appeal needs to include a severe threat, evidence suggesting that the target is especially vulnerable to the threat, and solutions that are easy to perform and effective. It should be noted, however, that fear appeals do not work in all circumstances. It is necessary to take account of the age of the target audience and the likelihood of voluntary message processing.

More generally, Witte (1995) has advocated a Persuasive Health Message Framework (PHM) based on elements from the Theory of Reasoned Action (Azjen, 1988), the Elaboration Likelihood Model (Petty and Cacioppo, 1986) and Protection Motivation Theory (Rogers, 1975). Witte argued that a persuasive health message should contain a threat message, an efficacy message, various cues, and that it should be targeted towards a specific award, regardless of the topic, type of message or environment. Thus, to motivate audiences into action, the message needs to convince individuals that they are susceptible to a severe threat and that adopting an easy and feasible recommended response would effectively avert the threat. In terms of types of specific arguments that can be used, Witte pointed out that these can either try to change beliefs, reinforce existing beliefs or introduce new beliefs. He noted that it is far easier to introduce, reinforce or build on existing beliefs in a health campaign than it is to try to change existing and entrenched beliefs. Thus the best campaigns are those that are framed to fit within acceptable beliefs and behaviours.

In terms of age, health campaigns are increasingly targeting children younger than has been the norm in the past. As far as child health campaigns are concerned, Austin (1995) has suggested that, to be effective, strategies need to micro-target the needs and interests of children of different ages and in different environments. They must also provide consistent messages from a variety of sources and over an extended period of time. Finally, they must emphasize giving children control and ownership of their own health decisions. Campaigns based on moralizing, scare tactics and knowledge-only approaches tend to be less effective with children. Rather, it is necessary to understand and respect the child's perspective, and how the problem relates to the child's resources, needs, goals and conflicting interests. Austin (1995) noted that children of different ages are motivated by different things and are particularly influenced by different information sources. Thus, children under the age of 5, tend to be motivated by tangible rewards from others and the avoidance of punishment, and find all information sources credible. Those between the age of 5 and 7 are motivated by rewards, moral labels and conventional rules, and find most sources of information credible. Children aged between 7 and 10 are motivated by social norms and the need for acceptance, and are particularly influenced by school, family and peers. Finally, older children are motivated by physical attractiveness and social power, and are most influenced by everyday role models and peers.

Ethical issues in disseminating health information to the wider public

It should be no surprise that working to improve the health of the public, irrespective of the age of the target audience, is likely to involve ethical value judgements. In the previous chapter we considered four basic principles that are used to guide health professionals' decisions. These principles (respect for autonomy, non-maleficence or doing no harm, beneficence or doing good, and justice) are also key to ethical health promotion. A higher-order principle that is often applied in relation to health promotion is that professionals should act in ways such that the benefits of any action will outweigh any disadvantages. However, the application of this principle can create conflict with the other principles. Thus, the introduction of smoking bans in public places is argued to offer the greatest benefit for the largest number of people, but can also directly conflict with the principle of autonomy when it comes to looking at the rights of individual smokers. The issues are even more complex when it comes to areas of health such as vaccination and screening programmes. Again, these can be well justified in terms of doing the greatest amount of good for the largest number of people, but may not be in the best interests of every individual child or parent. Freed et al. (2004) pointed out that, in the USA, most family physicians and almost all paediatricians reported at least one vaccine refusal from parents in 2000. Such refusal is likely to be exacerbated by the dissemination of information (and misinformation) and anecdotal reports by the media and the Internet of alleged vaccine reactions (Kimmel and Wolfe, 2005).

These ethical issues are addressed in the UK government's recent White Paper on public health (Department of Health, 2004). In the introduction to the paper, UK Health Minister, John Reid, stated that while we respect an individual's right to make their own choices, we need to respond to public concern that some people's choices can have a dangerous effect on other people's health. We therefore need to strike the right balance between allowing people to decide their own actions, while not allowing these actions to unduly inconvenience or damage the health of others.

The ethical principle of justice, or fairness for all, is particularly relevant in the area of health promotion, as decisions usually need to be made about allocating limited resources between different individuals and sectors of the population. Thus, in the previous chapter, we considered whether, in the case of screening, a less effective procedure for a relatively common condition should take priority (when resources are limited) over a very effective procedure for a much rarer condition. In order to weigh the potential benefits of any health programme against the risks, a distinction can be made between cost–benefit analysis and cost-effectiveness analysis (BMA, 1990). In the former case, a decision is typically whether to spend money to save lives, that is, to attempt to weigh lives against sums of money. In contrast, cost-effectiveness analysis makes the assumption that resources are available, even if limited, and is used to determine how best to limit any risks. As the BMA (1990) noted, given that risks to health may either relate to length of life or to quality of life, there is interest in making rationing fairer by combining these elements to produce an overall measure of benefit.

Summary

This chapter has looked at communication issues in relation to health promotion and disseminating information to the wider public. It started by considering what is involved in health promotion and then looked at health promotion in schools and the workplace. We next looked at three general strategies or approaches to health promotion and then considered in more detail three different channels (Patient Information Leaflets, the media and the Internet) that are commonly used to disseminate information to the wider public. Finally, we considered some ethical issues that arise in relation to health promotion and communicating health information to the general population.

Communication skills training

In several of the earlier chapters in this book we have noted the importance of healthcare professionals having good communication skills. There is now a large body of empirical evidence to show that healthcare providers who communicate well with patients make more accurate and complete diagnoses, are more likely to detect distress in patients and have patients who are more satisfied and less anxious. Their patients are also more likely to follow recommended advice and treatments, and have improved health indices and recovery rates (e.g. Di Blasi et al., 2001; Dulmen and Bensing, 2001; Fallowfield et al., 2002; Williams et al., 1998). Conversely, there is also evidence to show that poor communication between health professionals and patients can result in a number of negative health outcomes (e.g. MacDonald, 2004). Unfortunately, the manner of communication between doctors and patients is still a major cause of patient dissatisfaction (e.g. Roberts et al., 2001). Interestingly, most complaints about doctors concern poor communication and failure to listen, rather than competence or more technical aspects of consultations.

We also noted in Chapter 1 that poor communication between health-care providers and patients is often the result of inadequate training in communication skills. Somewhat surprisingly, an individual doctor may carry out between 150 000 and 200 000 patient interviews during the course of his or her career, but very few have received any formal training in communication, and much of the training that has been provided has been inadequate. The UK Health Services Commissioner's Annual Report (1993) noted that one reason for the inadequate training was that communication tends to be relegated to the hidden curriculum, rather than being formally and explicitly addressed. As Sleight (1995) pointed out, however, teaching communication skills is arguably one of the most important parts of the medical curriculum, and should not be considered to be an optional extra. Fortunately, there is now a growing body of empirical evidence to suggest that the provision of formal communication skills can significantly improve the quality of communications between healthcare providers and patients.

Chapter 5 included a number of useful guidelines for healthcare professionals when dealing with particular sub-groups of the population (such as older adults, children and parents, different ethnic groups and withdrawn or aggressive patients). Similarly, Chapter 6 included guidelines to help healthcare professionals to communicate complex risk information or bad news to patients or others. Many of these guidelines are likely to be incorporated into current communication skills training programmes. In addition, such programmes might also cover tips for how to increase the likelihood of particular aspects of the environment facilitating communication (as outlined in Chapter 2). The present chapter supplements the information that has already been covered in these earlier chapters. It starts by considering the different communication skills that are typically targeted in training programmes, including a number of the more basic skills, as well as the more complex skills needed for managing and resolving conflict in healthcare settings. It then looks at a number of different approaches to the provision of training. Finally, it reviews much of the empirical evidence from studies that have evaluated the success of existing programmes.

Basic communication skills

Communicating effectively with others requires the skilled use of various different techniques. In healthcare situations, the most commonly employed communication skills are questioning (including carrying out the 'medical' interview), explaining and providing information, listening, reinforcement and reflection, as well as being able to open and close interactions satisfactorily. Many of these skills include both verbal and non-verbal aspects, and communication skills training now routinely covers both the verbal and non-verbal components. These basic communication techniques will now be discussed in more detail.

Questioning

Questions are verbal statements, or non-verbal acts, that invite a answer (Stewart and Cash, 2000). We noted in Chapter 2 that to ask a question is one of the most powerful tools in communication (Hawkins and Power, 1999), as questions are at the heart of most interpersonal interactions. Clearly, the ability to ask questions effectively is a core skill for most health professionals, as they need to be able to ascertain certain basic information from patients and others before they can begin to make a diagnosis or give advice. Questions serve a number of different purposes, including opening discussions, obtaining information, assessing a patient's condition, diagnosing what is likely to be wrong and determining the most appropriate treatment or follow-up course of action. They can also be used to elicit the patient's attitudes and feelings, demonstrate interest and maintain control of the interaction.

As we noted in Chapter 2, there are two basic types of question. Open questions (such as 'what is the problem?') encourage longer unstructured answers. Clearly, these allow patients to say what is wrong with them in their own words, and discuss how they feel about it, but can result in irrelevant information being introduced into discussions. In contrast, closed questions (such as, 'have you been taking your medication?') typically encourage short yes/no responses. Closed questions are most useful for obtaining a limited amount of factual information in a limited time, or when it is necessary to obtain specific information which the patient has not provided. However, it must be recognized that the information elicited will depend on the specific questions asked, and may lead to the patient feeling frustrated as they have had little opportunity to express their own concerns and feelings. A number of studies have shown that healthcare providers tend to overuse closed questions (presumably to reduce the length of consultations), and often need training to use more open questions. In practice, most healthcare inter-actions will benefit from the use of a combination of open and closed questions. Whatever combination is decided on, overly complex questions (that often contain two or more sub-questions) and leading questions (that bias people towards responding in a particular way) should be avoided. Thus, a leading question, such as 'how beneficial did you find the medicine?' should be rephrased, or preceded by the more neutral question, 'has the medicine had any effect?'

The 'medical interview'

Much of the question asking that takes place in healthcare interactions will occur in the context of what is known as 'the medical interview'. Such interviews take place in many different settings, such as on hospital wards, in clinics, in GP surgeries and in community pharmacies. Whatever the particular setting, it is preferable to use quiet, private and comfortable conditions, with an appropriate seating arrangement (with the health profes-sional facing the patient). Lloyd and Bor (1996) outlined a number of guide-lines for conducting interviews. In terms of starting the interview, they suggested that patients should be greeted by name and asked to sit down. The healthcare professional should introduce themselves and explain the purpose of the interview, the need to take notes, and the attendance of others if relevant. During the main part of the interview, the professional should try to maintain a positive atmosphere, warm manner and good eye contact, should use open questions at the beginning, switching to specific closed questions when needed, and should listen carefully. While doing this they should be alert and responsive to both verbal and non-verbal cues that are emitted by the patient, and should facilitate the patient's input by using appropriate verbal and non-verbal responses themselves. At the end of the interview the professional should summarize what the patient has said and check that their understanding is accurate, ask them if there is anything that has been missed, and thank the patient. If relevant, they should explain what will happen next.

Explaining and providing information

Information provision serves a number of different purposes. Thus, information may be provided to help the patient understand what is wrong with them and how it might be treated, to reduce their uncertainty and anxiety, to correct mistaken beliefs, to give advice and to gain their co-operation in their healthcare management. Clearly, the way in which information is provided or explained can have a major effect on several aspects of patient care. As we have seen earlier in this book, a number of studies have shown that people who are provided with more, relevant, information often have higher levels of satisfaction, feel less anxious, experience less pain, are more adherent and have other improved health outcomes (e.g. Culos-Reed et al., 2000; Roter, 2000; Roter et al., 2001). Unfortunately, studies have also shown that healthcare providers are often not very good at providing the information that patients most want (e.g. Donovan and Blake, 1992; Noble, 1998; Williams, 1993). Indeed, failure to give adequate information or provide an adequate level of explanation has been noted to be one of the most common causes of dissatisfaction among patients (Berry, 2004; Luker et al., 1997).

As noted by Lloyd and Bor (1996), to provide information effectively, healthcare professionals need to be able to fully understand the information themselves and to convey it accurately, using ideas and language that will be easily understood by the patient. They also need to be prepared to respond to the recipient's questions and emotional reactions, and to tailor future information accordingly. Lloyd and Bor (1996) outlined a number of guidelines for healthcare professionals in relation to providing information to patients. These include describing the information that will be given, summarizing their understanding of the patient's problems, ascertaining the patient's understanding of their condition, using appropriate language, giving the most important information first, exploring the patient's views on information given, checking their understanding and negotiating future management of their care. In addition, Dickson et al. (1997) proposed that professionals should speak fluently, reduce vagueness, use examples and structure information effectively. In addition, they should use pauses appropriately, provide emphasis, and be expressive where appropriate.

As noted in Chapter 6, one difficult situation where information has to be provided is when healthcare providers have to break bad news to patients or relatives. It is clearly a matter of judgement and experience as to how bad news should best be broken, and each case may well need to be treated differently. A number of specific guidelines were outlined in Chapter 6.

Attending and listening

According to Burnard (1997), listening and attending are by far the most important aspect of being a healthcare professional. Attending is the act of focusing on the other person, what they are saying and what they are trying to communicate. Listening, in turn, is the process of 'hearing' the other person; not just what they say but how they say it and what other signals they convey. According to Burnard, it involves focusing on the actual words that clients use, the associated paralinguistics and the accompanying non-verbal behaviours. As noted in Chapter 2, the latter can sometimes portray contrary (and often more accurate) indications of the client's true feelings. Despite being one of the most central components of the communication process, effective or active listening can be one of the most difficult skills to acquire (Lloyd and Bor, 1996). It is not only important to listen, but to let the speaker know that you are listening carefully to them (that is, to show active listening). This can be done by using verbal and non-verbal signals (such as head nodding), appropriate follow-on questions, and reinforcement and reflection where relevant, and by summarizing and checking information and taking notes.

Wolff et al. (1983) suggested a number of guidelines that could be used to facilitate effective listening. These are:

1 Do not stereotype the speaker
2 Avoid distractions
3 Arrange a conducive environment
4 Be psychologically prepared to listen
5 Keep an open, analytical mind, searching for the central thrust of the speaker's message
6 Identify supporting arguments and facts
7 Do not dwell on one or two aspects at the expense of others
8 Delay judgement or refutation until you have heard the entire message
9 Do not formulate the next question while the speaker is relaying information
10 Be objective.

More recently, Egan (1998) suggested that use of the acronym SOLER could help healthcare providers to remember the key behaviours that can encourage active listening. These are sitting Squarely in relation to the client, maintaining an Open position, Leaning slightly forwards towards the client, maintaining reasonable Eye contact and Relaxing (and encouraging the client to relax).

Effective listening is necessary to gain a full and accurate understanding of the patient's problem and associated feelings, to communicate interest and concern, to encourage openness and to develop a more non-directive patient-centred style of interaction (Dickson et al., 1997). Buckman (1992) summarized the main benefits of effective listening as improved satisfaction, increased perceived competence of the healthcare provider and enhanced compliance with the treatment plan.

Reinforcement

It is a basic principle governing behaviour that people are more likely to do things that are associated with positive valued outcomes, and that are positively reinforced. Indeed, as a social skill, reinforcement is central to interpersonal interaction. As noted by Dickson et al. (1997), the use of social reinforcement serves a number of different purposes. Thus, it encourages the involvement of the other person, demonstrates interest, helps to develop and maintain relationships, provides reassurance, conveys warmth and helps to control the flow of conversation. The key behavioural components of reinforcement include acknowledgement, confirmation, paying compliments and making supportive and evaluative comments. Healthcare providers should use such behaviours where appropriate, to reinforce positive behaviours in patients and others.

Reflecting

This typically involves the healthcare professional rewording and feeding back the main elements of the patient's preceding comments. This can involve paraphrasing factual content, as well as trying to reflect feelings by demonstrating an understanding of them. Specifically, according to Dickson et al. (1997), reflection involves:

- recalling and restating the speaker's message correctly
- identifying the main factual and/or feeling aspects being expressed
- translating these into one's own words
- reflecting the essence of these facts and feelings without adding one's own interpretations
- checking the accuracy of reflection by monitoring the other person.

The key functions of reflection are to demonstrate interest and involvement, to use a patient-centred approach, to check for accuracy of understanding, to highlight certain facets of the patient's communication, to show respect for patients and their concerns, and to demonstrate empathy with the patient and their situation. Dickson et al suggested that, when using reflection, it is important to be accurate, concise and specific, to avoid interpreting people's statements (as opposed to rephrasing them) and to refrain from using stereotyped responses.

Opening and closing interactions

In terms of opening skills, it is well known that initial impressions have a large influence on the course, and success, of subsequent interactions. They frequently determine the length, tone and quality of first, and often follow-on, encounters. It only takes a few seconds to make an initial impression but the effects can be very long-lasting. At the start of interviews, or consultations, it is important for healthcare professionals to explain the purpose of the coming discussion and to give reasons for why particular information is being sought. They should then explain what the patient is expected to do and ascertain if the patient has any initial concerns. Interestingly, Davis and Fallowfield (1994) found that one of the main deficiencies of health professionals was their failure to greet patients appropriately and to introduce themselves and explain the purpose of the consultation. Similarly, Maguire et al. (1986), in their study of the communication skills of young doctors, reported that few explained the intended purpose of the interaction and the time available.

As far as closing skills are concerned, professionals need to arrange for a smooth and effective closure to interactions. This involves the use of techniques such as summarizing, checking understanding, discussing follow-up actions, using motivation and reinforcement, and asking if anything has been missed. It is also often appropriate to use non-task statements (such as asking about holidays), as well as to thank the patient and to say goodbye. Closing consultations can sometimes be difficult as what needs to be said will depend on the content of the preceding interaction, and will involve the patients' (at least tacit) agreement. Some patients have a tendency to introduce new information at, what doctors thought was, the end of the consultation. Such tendencies can be avoided, or at least reduced, if patients are encouraged to contribute fully earlier in the consultation.

Managing conflict

In addition, to covering these basic communication techniques, communication skills training also typically includes teaching healthcare professionals to deal with, and manage, conflict. It is not surprising that there is a potential for conflict in many healthcare situations. People are often placed in unfamiliar settings, in stressful and uncertain circumstances. In addition, many are in physical pain and are scared or apprehensive. Some healthcare professionals may be defensive or not sufficiently skilled at imparting difficult news and handling difficult people. Communication is central to conflict. It can be a causal factor, it is the primary means by which conflict is expressed and it can be used to manage and resolve conflict.

A number of different approaches to conflict have been identified (e.g. Northouse and Northouse, 1998). The least effective approach, or strategy, is the 'lose–lose strategy'. Although people do not usually intentionally adopt this approach, they can end up in this situation as a result of ineffective handling of conflict. Lose–lose situations come about because both participants try to dominate the other, and try to 'win all', but this usually results in both ending up losing. Another unsatisfactory approach is known as the 'win–lose strategy'. This approach comes about when one participant tries to take control over the other in order to 'win all'. However, even if the person is successful it means that the second person 'loses all', which is not usually a desirable outcome. It is therefore generally agreed that the most optimal approach to conflict resolution is the 'win–win strategy'. Unlike the other two approaches, this strategy allows both participants to feel that they have been successful, at least to some extent. This ideal strategy, and end result, however, are not always easy to achieve. They involve people putting their own position clearly, while at the same time listening to, and appreciating, the other person's position. They may require creative problem solving in trying to find a novel solution that allows both parties to come away from the situation feeling satisfied.

In addition, to these higher-level strategies, people approach interpersonal conflict using different styles of interaction. Northouse and Northouse (1998) identified the five main styles as follows:

1 *Avoidance.* This tends to be used by passive, unassertive people. It is rarely successful as most conflict does not go away if you simply ignore it. Avoiding conflict often leads to anxiety and stress, as well as to frustration and anger in others.
2 *Competition.* This style of interaction tends to be used by people who are very assertive and competitive. Again, it tends not to be a particularly effective approach to resolving conflict, as it does not allow for negotiation or compromise.
3 *Accommodation.* According to Northouse and Northouse (1998), accommodation is a conflict style that is 'unassertive but co-operative' (p. 247), as well as being 'other directed'. Although accommodation can be useful in some situations, it often results in one or other person just giving in to another.
4 *Compromise.* This fourth style includes an element of accommodation but also an element of competition. Although it can be successful, it often leads to both parties coming away from the situation feeling partly satisfied but partly dissatisfied. By going for a compromise solution they fail to achieve a more creative solution that could have resulted in a 'win–win' outcome.
5 *Collaboration.* The final approach identified by Northouse and Northouse (1998) is believed to be the most preferred style, although perhaps the most difficult to achieve. It requires both assertiveness and co-operation, as well as a lot of effort on behalf of the participants. If successful,

however, it should result in an effective solution to conflict where both parties leave the situation feeling fully satisfied.

In addition to outlining the different advantages and disadvantages of different strategies and styles of handling conflict, communication skills training will also try to teach simple methods that can be learned and applied to help manage the situation. For example, professionals may be taught to try to break down a conflict situation into small contributing elements, and then to address them individually. Training may also cover the need to define and clarify one's own position in an attempt to reduce misunderstanding.

Conflict can also arise in small-group situations, as a result of different participants having different (clashing) goals and styles of interaction. Hargie and Dickson (2004) outlined four key tactics that should be included in communication skills training aimed at handling conflict in small-group settings. These are:

♦ focusing on issues, rather than personalities
♦ making all contributors feel that their suggestions have, at least, some merit
♦ highlighting broad areas of agreement if these can be identified
♦ emphasizing 'we' and 'us' in order to try to establish or re-establish a stronger sense of 'group'.

Different approaches to communication skills training

A number of different approaches to communicate skills training have been identified. Dickson et al. (1997) listed the main four as being: doing the job, modelling the master, directed training and doing-based training.

Doing the job

This is the method that has been traditionally used by health professionals. It simply involves junior staff picking up knowledge about how to improve skills, while actually interacting with patients. However, the method is limited as the learning is predominantly by trial and error, and the learner may simply develop strategies for 'how to get through' the interaction, or to survive, rather than acquire more situationally appropriate skills.

Model the master

This is the classic apprenticeship model which involves observing a 'master' or more experienced colleague at work. It was assumed until relatively recently that students can acquire good communication skills by 'a sort of osmosis', by watching and modelling the behaviour of others. A weakness of this approach, however, is that it tends to lead to conservatism rather than innovation. The learner is unlikely to end up being more skilled than the master, and may pick up the master's mistakes and weaknesses.

Directed training

This tends to be the traditional didactic, or classroom-based approach, and is often more 'thinking' or intellectually based. Its chief weakness is that learning takes place 'out of context' and any skills acquired may not be applied in practice and may not be generalized to other appropriate situations.

Doing-based training

This final approach relies on action as a means of bringing about learning. The trainee attempts the skill and is given feedback on their performance by the trainer or other observers. The feedback is then used to improve their subsequent performance.

According to Dickson et al. (1997), in most situations, it is best to use a combination of different approaches, rather than just a single method. This may, for example, involve one or two initial classroom sessions, followed by the use of the final method so that the trainee can learn to apply the skills that have been taught and receive feedback and further guidance while doing so. Maguire et al. (1989) suggested that the key elements in any training package include the learner being given written instructions about the skills to be used, opportunity to practise the skills with real or simulated patients under controlled conditions, and feedback on their performance, preferably by using an audio-or video-taped replay. They should also be able to discuss the observed performance with their trainer to obtain any necessary clarifications. Similarly, Leigh and Reiser (1986) advocated that training will be most successful if skills are taught in situations that mirror the situation in which they will be used in practice. They suggested that training that uses direct supervised contact with patients, in which the student receives good feedback immediately after the interaction, should work best.

Empirical evaluation of communication skills training

A number of researchers and practitioners have proposed that healthcare professionals can be taught to use patient-centred communication skills (e.g. Langewitz et al., 1998). It has also been noted that this approach may be particularly effective when having to interact with difficult people or in difficult circumstances (e.g. Anderson and Sharpe, 1991; Sharpe et al., 1994). In line with this, Forshaw (2002) argued that it is relatively easy to teach professionals to use some very basic rules that will improve their communications, such as greeting patients by name, explaining the purpose of procedures, using more direct eye contact and thanking patients at the end of a consultation. All of these contribute to positive relationship building and effective interactions.

In a relatively early study, Maguire et al. (1986) found that students who received formal feedback-based training showed significant improvements in their communication skills. Specifically, compared with a control group, the feedback-trained group obtained three times more relevant and accurate information about the patient's problem, and were given higher ratings by patients. In addition, in follow-up studies, they were found to be more empathic and more self-assured when interviewing patients, and more likely to use an open style of questioning and to show appropriate responding to patient cues.

More recently, Fallowfield and colleagues have carried out a series of studies that have applied, and evaluated the effectiveness of, formal communication skills training. Fallowfield et al. (2002), for example, conducted a study to assess the efficacy of an intensive three-day training course on communication skills, using a randomized control trial. The participants in the study were 160 oncologists, recruited from 34 UK cancer centres. They were given one of four different treatments: written feedback alone, course alone, written feedback followed by the course, or no training (the control condition). The course was designed specifically for oncologists and was based on one used extensively in the USA. The focus was user centred and it incorporated cognitive, affective and behavioural components. It involved participants interacting with trained 'simulated patients' and receiving feedback on their performance. At each of two different assessment periods, consultations with 6 to 10 consecutive 'patients' per doctor were videotaped. A total of nearly 2500 patients participated in the study. The investigators used a mixture of objective and subjective post-training performance measures, with ratings being made by researchers, doctors and patients. There were additional analyses based on length and content of the interaction. The primary outcomes were objective improvements following the training in key communication skills such as showing empathy, responding appropriately to patient cues and asking appropriate questions. Overall, it was found that course attendance significantly improved performance in terms of these primary outcomes, but there was little evidence for the effectiveness of written feedback. There was also evidence that the improvements persisted with time. Fallowfield et al. (2003) conducted a follow-up study and found that 12 to 15 months post-intervention, there was still an enduring effect of communication skills training, with virtually no attrition in improved skill use. There was also evidence for appropriate transfer into the clinic. In addition, some new skills that were not apparent in the initial phase of the study (such as making fewer interruptions and increased use of summarization of information) emerged in the follow-up study.

In looking at the effectiveness of different training programmes, Cegala and Broz (2003) noted that there is now considerable evidence that the provision of training in communication skills is effective. However, they warned that it needs to be recognized that around 30 per cent of the studies reviewed by them had relied solely, or primarily, on participants' self-perception or self-evaluation of their communication competence. Although self-perceptions are often related to actual performance, they should not be used as sole evidence for evaluating the effectiveness of training programmes. Cegala and Broz also noted that very few programmes have assessed the longer-term effects of training. A strength of the Fallowfield et al study, described earlier, is that it used a combination of subjective and objective measures, and that it also included a follow-on assessment phase.

Given the increased recognition of the value of communication skills training, many medical schools now routinely incorporate it into their curricula. Haq et al. (2004) described a programme in the USA (Undergraduate Medical Education for the 21st Century – UME-21) to co-ordinate the skills training that is provided for medical students. In the 12 participating medical schools, curricula themes included conflict resolution, delivery of bad news, addressing preferences for end-of-life care, health education, and working effectively with families and with patients from diverse backgrounds. The acquired skills were assessed through structured clinical examinations, focused observation and feedback, and debriefing sessions based on videotapes. Haq et al reported that the results of the formal assessments showed beneficial effects of the skills training in the students. Clearly, however, it is not known whether the acquired skills will be incorporated into routine practice once the students have qualified.

Communication skills training for patients

Another concern raised by Cegala and Broz (2003) is that there has been relatively little research on the effectiveness of patient- (as opposed to provider-) based training. Most of the studies that have been conducted with patients have centred on providing training on information seeking, provision and verification. Cegala and Broz noted that, to date, the impact of training on question-asking has been quite modest, with around half of the studies reporting positive effects. The most positive gains have come from studies that have included a practice component, and/or have tailored the content and training objectives to patient needs (see also Kreuter et al., 2000). Finally, Cegala and Broz pointed out that virtually no research has looked at the training of both providers and patients in order to examine and improve interactive contributions. Similarly, there is still very little known about how individual differences such as gender, ethnicity and educational background interact with skills training.

As far as patient training is concerned, Post et al. (2002) carried out a review of randomized control trials that had taken place in an outpatient setting between 1975 and 2000, and that had involved teaching patients to communicate with physicians. Patient communication interventions were classified as being either high, medium or low intensive, depending on the length of the intervention, as well as in terms of the use of personnel and the estimated cost. Thus, for example, a high-intensive intervention might have involved face-to-face training, conducted by a research assistant for 15 minutes before a scheduled appointment. In contrast, a low-intensive intervention might have involved simply giving patients a blank sheet of paper and getting them to write down three questions that they would like to ask the doctor. The results of the review showed that skills training resulted in patient improvement on a variety of outcomes. Positive change variables included improved communication, medical outcomes, functional status and adherence to treatment. Patient communication training changed the nature of the physician–patient interaction, with patients exhibiting and feeling increased control. However, the studies revealed mixed findings in terms of effects on patient satisfaction. In addition, Post et al noted that, overall, there was a wide variation in the types of study design used, the type of intervention and outcomes, and that this hindered the ability to draw well-founded conclusions.

Harrington et al. (2004) carried out a more recent review of intervention studies that have focused on improving patients' communications with their doctors. The review covered a total of 20 studies, half of which were randomized control trials. These authors found that, overall, half of the interventions resulted in increased patient participation, with there being a greater increase in requests for clarification than in question asking. There were significant improvements in perceptions of control over health, preferences for taking an active role in healthcare, recall of information, adherence to recommendations, attendance and clinical outcomes. As with the Post et al review, there were relatively few significant improvements in patient satisfaction. Clearly, there is much more to be done in this important area.

Summary

This final chapter has emphasized the importance of healthcare professionals having good communication skills, and has shown that such skills can be explicitly trained. It has also acknowledged the increasing recognition of this by government, the 'medical establishment' and others. The chapter then looked at some of the core skills that are needed for effective communication, as well as how best to manage and resolve conflict. Finally, we reviewed a number of the empirical studies that have assessed the effects of communication skills training in healthcare professionals and patients. Although there is still much more to do in this important area, the preliminary indications are very positive.

Throughout this book, I have stressed the importance of *effective* communication in health. We have seen some of the negative outcomes of poor communication, and have discussed a number of the common problem areas. We have also identified a number of basic and more complex communication skills that contribute to effective (and less effective) interactions with others. In this final chapter, we have evaluated evidence to show that the effective use of such skills can be explicitly trained. Hopefully, the increasing recognition, availability and use of such training should result in more effective health communication between the different players in the healthcare process in the years to come.

LIBRARY, UNIVERS   CHESTE

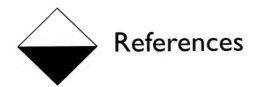# References

Adelman, R.D., Greene, M.G. and Charon, R. (1991). Issues in physician–elderly patient interaction, *Ageing and Society*, 11, 127–48.

Albert, T. and Chadwick, S. (1992). How readable are practice leaflets? *British Medical Journal*, 305, 1266–8.

Armitage, C.J. and Conner, M. (2000). Attitudinal ambivalence: a test of three key hypotheses, *Personality and Social Psychology Bulletin*, 26, 1421–32.

Anderson, L.A. and Sharpe, P.A. (1991). Improving patient and provider communication: a synthesis and review of communication interventions, *Patient Education & Counselling*, 17, 99–134.

Austin, E.W. (1995). Reaching young audiences; developmental considerations in designing health messages, in E. Maibach and R.L. Parrot (eds), *Designing Health Messages: Approaches from Communication Theory and Public Health Practice*. Thousand Oaks, CA: Sage.

Azjen, I. (1985). From intentions to action: a theory of planned behaviour, in J. Kuhl and J. Beckman (eds), *Action Control: From Cognitions to Behaviors*. New York: Springer Verlag.

Azjen, I. (1988). *Attitudes, Personality and Behaviour*. Milton Keynes: Open University Press.

Barlow, J.H. and Wright, C.C. (1998). Knowledge in patients with rheumatoid arthritis: a longer term follow-on of a randomised control study of patient education leaflets, *British Journal of Rheumatology*, 37, 373–6.

Baylav, A. (1996). Overcoming culture and language barriers, *Practitioner*, 250, 403–6.

BBC (2005a). BBC health conditions: dementia, www.bbc.co.uk/health/conditions/dementia/shtml.

BBC (2005b). BBC News, Education, England's staggering adult illiteracy, http//news.bbc.co.uk/1/hi/education/302972.stm.

Beauchamp, T. and Childress, J. (1994). *Principals of Biomedical Ethics*, 4th edn. Oxford: Oxford University Press.

Becker, M.H. and Rosenstock, I.M. (1984). Compliance with medical advice, in A. Steptoe and A. Mathews (eds), *Healthcare and Human Behaviour*. London: Academic Press.

Beckman, H.B. and Frankel, R.M. (1984). The effect of physician behaviour on the collection of data, *Annals of Internal Medicine*, 101, 692–6.

Bennett, P. (1998). *Communicating about Risks to Public Health: Pointers to Good Practice*. London: Department of Health.

Bennett, P. and Murphy, S. (1997). *Psychology and Health Promotion*. Buckingham: Open University Press.

Bensing, J.M. and Verhaak, P.F.M. (2004). Communication in medical encounters: towards a health psychology perspective, in A. Kaptein and J. Weinman (eds), *Health Psychology: An Introduction*. Oxford: Blackwell.

Bental, D.S., Cawsey, A. and Jones, B. (1999). Patient information systems that tailor to the individual, *Patient Education and Counselling*, 36, 171–90.

Berg, J.W., Appelbaum, P.S., Parker, L.S. and Lidz, C.W. (2001). *Informed Consent: Legal Theory and Clinical Practice*. New York: Oxford University Press.

Berger, C. (1995). A plan based approach to strategic communication, in D. Hewes (ed.), *The Cognitive Basis of Interpersonal Communication*. Hillsdale, NJ: Lawrence Erlbaum Associates.

Berland, G., Elliott, M., Algazy, J., Kravitz, R. et al. (2001). Health information on the Internet: accessibility, quality and readability in English and Spanish, *Journal of the American Medical Association*, 285, 2612–21.

Berne, E. (1958). Transactional analysis: an effective method of group therapy, *American Journal of Psychotherapy*, 12, 735–43.

Bernhardt, J.M. and Cameron, K.A. (2003). Accessing, understanding and applying health communication messages: the challenge of health literacy, in T.L. Thompson, A.M. Dorsey, K.I. Miller and R. Parrott (eds), *Handbook of Health Communication*. Mahwah, NJ: Lawrence Erlbaum Associates.

Berry, D.C. (2004). *Risk Communication and Health Psychology*. Milton Keynes: Open University Press.

Berry, D.C. (2006). Informing people about the risks and benefits of medicines: implications for the safe and effective use of medicinal products, *Current Drug Safety*, 1, 121–6.

Berry, D.C., Courtenay, M. and Bersellini, E. (2006). Attitudes towards, and information needs in relation to, nurse prescribing in the UK: an empirical study, *Journal of Clinical Nursing*, 15, 22–8.

Berry, D.C., Holden. W. and Bersellini, E. (2004). Interpretation of recommended risk terms: differences between doctors and lay people, *International Journal of Pharmacy Practice*, 12, 117–24.

Berry, D.C., Michas, I.C. and DeRosis, F. (1998). Evaluating explanations about drug prescriptions: effects of varying the nature of information about side effects and its relative position in explanations, *Psychology and Health*, 13, 767–84.

Berry, D.C., Raynor D.K. and Knapp, P.R. (2002). Provision of information about drug side-effects to patients, *Lancet*, 359, 853–4.

Berry, D.C., Raynor, D.K., Knapp, P.R. and Bersellini, E. (2003). Patient understanding of risk: impact of EU Guidelines and other risk scales for consumer medicines information, *Drug Safety*, 26, 1–11.

Bersellini, E. and Berry, D.C. (2004). Communicating information about medicines: the benefits of a benefit statement, *Proceedings of the British Psychological Society*, 12, 35.

Bersellini, E. and Berry, D.C. (in press). Benefits of providing benefit information:

examining the effectiveness of provision of simple benefit statements on people's judgements about a medicine, *Psychology & Health*.

Bibace, R. and Walsh, M.E. (1981). Developmental stages in children's conceptions of illness, in G.C. Stone, F. Cohen and N.E. Adler (eds), *Health Psychology: A Handbook*. San Francisco, CA: Jossey-Bass.

Biek, M., Wood, W. and Chaiken, S. (1996). Working knowledge, cognitive processing and attitudes: on the determinants of bias, *Personality and Social Psychology Bulletin*, 22, 547–56.

Bishop, P., Kirwan, J. and Windsor, K. (1996). *The ARC Patient Literature Evaluation Project*. Chesterfield: The Arthritis and Rheumatism Council.

Bloom, J.R. (1996). Social support of the cancer patient and the role of the family, in L. Baider, C.L. Cooper and A. Kaplan DeNour (eds), *Cancer and the Family*. New York: Wiley.

Bohner, G., Moskowitz, G.B. and Chaiken, S. (1995). The interplay of heuristic and systematic processing of social information, *European Review of Social Psychology*, 6, 33–68.

Bormann, E. (1990). *Small Group Communication: Theory and Practice*. New York: Harper and Row.

Brashers, D., Goldsmith, D. and Hsieh, E. (2002). Information seeking and avoiding in health contexts, *Human Communication Research*, 28, 258–71.

Bredin, M., Corner, J., Krishnasamy, M., Plant, H., Bailey, C. and O'Hearn, R. (1999). Multicentre randomised controlled trial of nursing intervention for breathlessness in patients with lung cancer, *British Medical Journal*, 318, 901–4.

Brilhart, J. and Galanes, G. (1998). *Group Discussion*, 9th edn. Boston, MA: McGraw-Hill.

British Medical Association (BMA) (1990). *The BMA Guide to Living with Risk*. London: Penguin.

Brookner, A. (1984). *Hotel du Lac*. London: Grafton Books.

Brooks, W. and Heath, R. (1993). *Speech Communication*. Dubuque, IA: W.C. Brown.

Brown, H., Ramchandani, M., Gillow, J. and Tsaloumas, M. (2004). Are patient information leaflets contributing to informed consent for cataract surgery?, *Journal of Medical Ethics*, 30, 218–20.

Brown, T.F., Massoud, E. and Bance, M. (2003). Informed consent in otologic surgery: prospective study of risk recall by patients and impact of written summaries of risk, *The Journal of Otolaryngology*, 32, 368–72.

Bryant, G.D. and Norman, G.R. (1980). Expressions of probability: words and numbers, *New England Journal of Medicine*, 302, 411.

Buckman, R. (1992). *How to Break Bad News: A Guide for Healthcare Professionals*. London: Macmillan.

Burnard, P. (1997). *Effective Communication Skills for Health Professionals*, 2nd edn. Cheltenham: Stanley Thornes.

Burton, G. and Dimbleby, R. (1995). *Between Ourselves: An introduction to Interpersonal Communication*. London: Arnold.

Bynner, J. and Parsons, S. (1997). *It Doesn't Get Any Better: The Impact of Poor Basic Skills on the Lives of 37 Year Olds*. London: The Basic Skills Agency.

Carlson, E.A., Li, S. and Holm, K. (1997). An analysis of menopause in the popular press, *Health Care for Women International*, 18, 557–64.

Cartwright, A. (1990). Medicine taking by people aged 65 or more, *British Medical Journal*, 46, 63–76.

Cassileth, B.R., Zupkis, R.V., Sutton-Smith, K. and March, V. (1980). Informed consent: why are its goals imperfectly realized?, *New England Journal of Medicine*, 302, 896–900.

Cegala, D.J. and Broz, S.L. (2003). Provider and patient communication skills training, in T.L. Thompson, A.M. Dorsey, K.I. Miller and R. Parrott (eds), *Handbook of Health Communication*. Mahwah, NJ: Lawrence Erlbaum Associates.

Centre for Health Quality Improvement (1997). *High Quality Matters*. Newsletter Issue 1. Winchester: Centre for Health Quality Improvement.

Chaiken, S. (1980). Heuristic versus systematic information processing and use of source vs message cues in persuasion, *Journal of Personality and Social Psychology*, 39, 752–66.

Chaiken, S. (1987). The heuristic model of persuasion, in M.P. Zanna, J.M. Olsen and C.P. Herman (eds), *Social Influence: The Ontario Symposium*, vol. 5. Hillsdale, NJ: Lawrence Erlbaum Associates.

Charles, C., Gafni, A. and Whelan, T. (1997). Shared decision-making in the medical encounter: what does it mean? (Or it takes at least two to tango), *Social Science and Medicine*, 44, 681–92.

Chrystal, D. (2005). *Pocket Quotations*. London: Penguin.

Claesson, S., Morrison, A., Wertheimer, A.I. and Berger, M.L. (1999). Compliance with prescription drugs: challenges for the elderly population, *Pharmacy World & Science*, 21, 256–9.

Clark, H.H. (1985). Language use and language users, in G. Lindzey and E. Aronson (eds), *Handbook of Social Psychology*. New York: Random House.

Clowers, M. (2000). Urban female teenagers' perceptions of medical communication, *Adolescence*, 35, 571–85.

Cole-Kelly, K. (1992). Illness stories and patient care in the family practice context, *Family Medicine*, 24, 45–8.

Corke, C., Stow, P., Green, D., Agar, J. and Henry, M. (2005). How do doctors discuss major interventions in high risk patients?, *British Medical Journal*, 330, 182.

Coudeyre, E., Poraudeau, S., Revel, M., Kahan, A., Drape, J.L. and Ravaud, P. (2002). Beneficial effects of information leaflets before spinal steroid injection, *Joint Bone Spine*, 69, 597–603.

Coulter, A. (1999). Paternalism or partnership? Patients have grown up – and there's no going back, *British Medical Journal*, 19, 719–20.

Coulter, A., Entwistle, V. and Gilbert, D. (1998). *Informing Patients: An Assessment of the Quality of Patient Information Materials*. London: King's Fund.

Craig, R. (1999). Communication theory as a field, *Communication Theory*, 9, 119–61.

Crawford, M.J., Rutter, D., Manley, C., Weaver, T., Bhui, K., Fulop, N. and Tyrer, P. (2002). Systematic review of involving patients in the planning and development of healthcare, *British Medical Journal*, 325, 1–5.

Cuervo, L.G. and Aronson, J.K. (2004). The road to healthcare, *British Medical Journal*, 329, 1–2.

Culos-Reed, S.N., Rejeski, W.J., McAuley, E., Ockene, J.K. and Roter, D.L. (2000). Predictors of adherence to behaviour change interventions in the elderly, *Controlled Clinical Trials*, 21, 200–5.

Curtis, J.R., Wenrich, M.D., Carline, J.D., Shannon, S.E., Ambrozy, D.M. and Ramsay, P.G. (2001). Understanding physicians' skills at providing end-of-life care perspectives of patients, families and healthcare workers, *Journal of General Internal Medicine*, 16, 41–9.

Danis, M. and Churchill, L.R. (1991). Autonomy and the common weal, *Hastings Centre Report*, 21, 25–31.

Davis, H. and Fallowfield, L. (1994). *Counselling and Communication in Healthcare*. Chichester: John Wiley.

Davis, T. and Wolf, M. (2004). Health literacy: implications for family medicine, *Family Medicine*, 36, 595–8.

De Jong, W., Franz, H.G., Wolfe, S.M., Nathan, H., Payne, D., Reitsma, W. and Beasley, C. (1998). Requesting organ donation: an interview study of donor and non-donor families, *American Journal of Critical Care*, 7, 13–23.

De Vito, J. (1998). *The Interpersonal Communication Book*, 8th edn. New York: Longman.

Delamothe, T. (1998). Who killed Cock Robin?, *British Medical Journal*, 316, 1757.

Department of Health (1992). *The Health of the Nation: A Summary of the Government's Proposals*. London: HMSO.

Department of Health (1999). *Saving Lives: Our Healthier Nation*. London: HMSO.

Department of Health (2001). *UK National Health Service Framework for Older People*. London: Department of Health.

Department of Health (2004). *Better Information, Better Choices, Better Health: Putting Information at the Centre of Care*. London: Department of Health.

Department of Health and Human Services (1996). Prescription drug information for patients: notice of request for collaboration to develop an action plan, *Federal Regulations*, 61, 43769–70.

Di Blasi, Z., Harkness, E., Ernst, E., Georgiou, A. and Kleijnen, J. (2001). Influence of context effects on health outcomes: a systematic review, *Lancet*, 357, 757–62.

Diaz, J.A., Griffith, R.A., Ng, J.J., Steven, M.D., Reinert, S.E., Friedmann, M.D. and Moulton, A.W. (2002). Patients' use of the Internet for medical information, *Journal of General Internal Medicine*, 17, 180–5.

Dickens B.M. and Cook R.J. (2004). Dimensions of informed consent to treatment, *International Journal of Gynecology & Obstetrics*, 85, 309–14.

Dickinson, D., Raynor, D.K. and Duman, M. (2001). Patient information leaflets for medicines: using consumer testing to determine the most effective design, *Patient Educational and Counselling*, 43, 147–59.

Dickson, D., Hargie, O. and Morrow, N. (1997). *Communication Skills Training for Health Professionals*. London: Chapman and Hall.

Doak, C.C., Doak, L.G., Friedell, G.H. and Meade, C.D. (1998). Improving comprehension for cancer patients with low literacy skills: strategies for clinicians, *CA – A Cancer Journal for Clinicians*, 48, 151–62.

Donovan, J.L. and Blake, D.R. (1992). Patient non-compliance: deviance or reasoned decision-making?, *Social Science and Medicine*, 34, 507–13.

Dorn, L.D. (1984). Children's concepts of illness: clinical applications, *Pediatric Nursing*, 10, 325–7.

Douglas, T. (2000). *Survival in groups*, 3rd edn. Buckingham: Open University Press.

Dowling, H. (1996). Consumer product information: where to from here?, *Australian Journal of Hospital Pharmacy*, 26, 293–8.

Doyal, L. (2001). Informed consent: moral necessity or illusion?, *Quality in Health Care*, 10, 29–33.

Dulmen, A.M. and Bensing, J.M. (2001). *The Effect of Context in Healthcare: A Programming Study*. The Hague: RGO.

Duxbury, J. (2000). *Difficult Patients*. Oxford: Butterworth-Heineman.

Edelmann, R.J. (2000). *Psychosocial Aspects of the Health Care Process*. London: Prentice Hall.

Edwards, I.R. and Hugman, B. (1997). The challenge of effectively communicating risk-benefit information, *Drug Safety*, 17, 216–27.

Edwards, M. (2004). Difficult conversations with children and parents, in E. MacDonald (ed.), *Difficult Conversations in Medicine*. Oxford: Oxford University Press.

Edwards, S.J.L, Lilford, R.J. and Hewison, J. (1998). The ethics of randomized controlled trials from the perspectives of patients, the public, and healthcare professionals, *British Medical Journal*, 317, 1209–12.

Egan, G. (1998). *The Skilled Helper*. London: Brooks Cole.

Eiser, C. and Twamley, S. (1999). Talking to children about health and illness, in M. Murray and K. Chamberlain (eds), *Qualitative Health Psychology*. London: Sage.

Ekman, P. (1982). *Emotion in the Human Face*. New York: Cambridge University Press.

Ekman, P. and Friesen, W. (1969). The repertoire of non-verbal behaviour: categories, origins, usage and coding, *Semiotica*, 1, 49–98.

Elder, M.J. and Suter, A. (2005). What do patients want to know before they have cataract surgery?, *British Journal of Ophthalmology*, 88, 1–3.

Eng, T.R. (2001). *The Health Landscape: A Terrain Map of Emerging Health Information and Communication Technologies in Health and Healthcare*. Princeton, NJ: Robert Wood Johnson Foundation.

Epstein, R.M., Campbell, T.L., Cohen-Cole, S.A., McWhinney, I.R. and Smilkstein, G. (1993). Perspectives on patient–doctor communication, *Journal of Family Practice*, 37, 377–88.

European Commission (1992). *EEC Directive 92/27/EEC on Labelling of Medicinal Products for Human Use and on Package Leaflets* (OJ No. L113 of 30 April 1992).

European Commission (1996). *Draft Guideline on the Readability of the Label and Package Leaflet of Medicinal Products for Human Use*. Brussels: European Commission.

European Commission (1998). *A Guideline on the Readability of the Label and Package Leaflet of Medicinal Products for Human Use*. Brussels: EC Pharmaceuticals Committee.

European Commission (2005). *Guidance Concerning 'Consultations with Target Patient Groups' for the Package Leaflet* (Directive 2004/27/EC). EC Pharmaceuticals, August.

Eysenbach, G. (2000). Consumer health informatics, *British Medical Journal*, 320, 1713–16.

Facts on Illiteracy in America (2005). http://Indian-river.fls.us/living/services/als/facts.html.

Fallowfield, L. (2002). Talking about difficult things in cancer: do we achieve what patients need?, *Drugs of Today*, 38, 79–87.

Fallowfield, L., Jenkins, V., Farewell, V., Saul, J., Duffy, A. and Eves, R. (2002). Efficacy of a cancer research UK communication skills training mode for oncologists: a random controlled trial, *Lancet*, 359, 650–6.

Fallowfield, L., Jenkins, V., Farewell, V. and Solis-Trapala, I. (2003). Enduring impact of communication skills training: results of a 12 month follow up, *British Journal of Cancer*, 89, 1445–9.

Farrell, G.A. and Gray, C. (1992). *Aggression: A Nurses' Guide to Therapeutic Management*. London: Scutari Press.

Federal Drug Administration (FDA) (2006). *Final Guidelines for Industry: Content and Format of Labelling for Human Prescription Drug and Biological Products*. US Food & Drug Administration, Department of Health and Human Sciences.

Federal Institute for Occupational Safety and Health (1996). European Network for Workplace Health Promotion. 1st Meeting of Member States. Report of workshop on 21 June 1995, in *Dortmund Conference Report Tb72*. NW Bremerhaven: Wirtschaftverlag.

Feld, A.D. (2004). Informed consent: not just for procedures anymore, *American Journal of Gastroenterology*, 99, 977–80.

Fletcher, C. (1980). Listening and talking to patients: some special problems, *British Medical Journal*, 281, 1056–8.

Fletcher, C. (1988). On truth telling, *Pharos Alpha Omega Alpha Honorary Medical Society*, 51, 37.

Fogel, J. (2003). Internet use for cancer information among racial/ethnic populations and low literacy groups, *Cancer Control*, 10, 45–51.

Forshaw, M. (2002). *Essential Health Psychology*. London: Arnold.

Fox, S. and Fallows, D. (2003). *Internet Health Resources: Half of American Adults Have Searched Online for 16 Health Topics Ranging from Disease Information to Smoking Cessation Strategies*. Washington, DC: The Pew Internet and American Life Project.

Fraser, C. and Burcell, B. (2001). *Introducing Social Psychology*. Cambridge: Polity Press.

Freed, G.L., Clark, S.J., Hobbs, B.F. and Santoli, J.M. (2004). Parental vaccine safety concerns: the experiences of paediatric and family physicians, *American Journal of Preventative Medicine*, 26, 11–14.

French, J.F. and Adams, L.A. (2002). From analysis to synthesis: theories of health education, in D.F. Marks (ed.), *The Health Psychology Reader*. London: Sage.

General Medical Council (GMC) (1993). *Tomorrow's Doctors: Recommendations on Undergraduate Medical Education*. London: General Medical Council.

General Medical Council (GMC) (1999). *Seeking Patients' Consent: The Ethical Considerations*. London: General Medical Council.

Gergen, K. and Gergen, M. (1988). Narrative and the self as relationship, in L. Berkowitz (ed.), *Advances in Experimental Social Psychology*, vol. 21. New York: Academic Press.

Gigerenzer, G. (2002). *Reckoning with Risk*. London: Penguin.

Glajchen, M., Fitzmartin, R.R., Blum, D. and Swanton, R. (1995). Psychosocial barriers to cancer pain relief, *Cancer Practice*, 3, 76–82.

Gortmaker, S.L., Beasley, C.L., Sheehy, E., Lucas, B.A., Brigham, L.E., Grenvik, A., Patterson, R.H., Garrison, N., McNamara, P. and Evanisko, M.J. (1998). Improving the request process to increase family consent for organ donation, *Journal of Transplant Coordination*, 8(4), 210–17.

Greenfield, S., Kaplan, S. and Ware, J.E. (1985). Expanding patient involvement in care: effects on patient outcomes, *Annals of Internal Medicine*, 102, 520–8.

Gross, T., Marguccio, I. and Martinoli, S. (2000). Attitudes of hospital staff involved in organ donation to the procedure, *Transplant International*, 13, 351–6.

Gurm, H.S. and Litaker, D.G. (2000). Framing procedural risks to patients: is 99% safe the same as a risk of 1 in 100?, *Academic Medicine*, 75, 840–2.

Hadlow, J. and Pitts, M. (1991). The understanding of common health terms by doctors, nurses and patients, *Social Science & Medicine*, 32, 193–6.

Hale, J.L. and Dillard, J.P. (1995). Fear appeals in health promotion campaigns: too much, too little or just right?, in E. Maibach and R.L. Parrott, R.L. (eds), *Designing Health Messages: Approaches from Communication Theory and Public Health Practice*. Thousand Oaks, CA: Sage.

Hall, J. (1996). Touch, status, and gender at professional meetings, *Journal of Nonverbal Behavior*, 20, 23–44.

Haq, C., Steele, D.J., Marchand, L., Seibert, C. and Brody, D. (2004). Integrating the art and science of medical practice: innovations in teaching medical communication skills, *Family Medicine*, 36, 43–50.

Hardey, M. (1999). Doctor in the house: the Internet as a source of lay health knowledge and the challenge to expertise, *Sociology of Health & Illness*, 21, 820–35.

Hargie, O. (1997). Interpersonal communication: a theoretical framework, in O. Hargie (ed.). *The Handbook of Communication Skills*, 2nd edn. London: Routledge.

Hargie, O. and Dickson, D. (2004). *Skilled Interpersonal Communication: Research, Theory and Practice*. Hove: Brunner Routledge.

Hargie, O. and Marshall, P. (1986). Interpersonal communication: a theoretical framework, in O. Hargie (ed.). *A Handbook of Communication Skills*. London: Croom Helm.

Hargie, O., Dickson, D., Boohan, M. and Hughes, K. (1998). A survey of communication skills training in UK schools of medicine: present practices and prospective proposals, *Medical Education*, 32, 25–34.

Harmsen, H., Meevswesen, L., Van Wieringen, J., Bernsen, R. and Bruijnzeels, M. (2003). When cultures meet in general practice: intercultural differences between GPs and parents of child patients, *Patient Education & Counselling*, 51, 99–106.

Harrington, J., Noble, L.M. and Newman, S.P. (2004). Improving patients' communication with doctors: a systematic review of intervention studies, *Patient Education & Counselling*, 52, 7–16.

Harrison, J.A., Mullen, P.D. and Green, L.W. (1992). A meta-analysis of studies of the Health Belief Model with adults, *Health Education Research*, 7, 107–16.

Hawkins, K. and Power, C. (1999). Gender differences in questions asked during small decision-making group discussions, *Small Group Research*, 30, 235–56.

Heath, R. and Bryant, J. (2000). *Human Communication Theory and Research: Concepts, Contexts and Challenges*. Mahwah, NJ: Lawrence Erlbaum Associates.

Heaven, C.M. (1997). The role of clinical supervision in communication skills training, unpublished PhD thesis, University of Manchester.

Hembroff, L.A., Holmes-Rovner, M. and Wills, C.E. (2004). Treatment decision-making and form of risk communication: results of a factorial survey, *BMC Medical Information Decision Making*, 4, 1–20.

Henley, N. (1973). The politics of touch, in P. Brown (ed.), *Radical Psychology*. New York: Harper and Row.

Hoffrage, U., Lindsey, S., Hertwig, R. and Gigerenza, G. (2000). Medicine: communicating statistical information, *Science*, 290, 2261–2.

Hollinger, L. and Buschmann, M. (1993). Factors influencing perception of touch by elderly nursing home residents and their health caregivers, *International Journal of Nursing Studies*, 30, 445–61.

Hollingshead, A.B. (1996). The rank order effect: decision procedure, communication technology and group decisions, *Organisational Behaviour and Human Decision Processes*, 68, 1–13.

Hollingshead, A.B. (1998). Retrieval processes in transactive memory systems, *Journal of Personality and Social Psychology*, 74, 659–71.

Horsch, B.M. and Harding, C. (1997). *The Intelligent Patient's Guide to the Doctor–Patient Relationship: Learning How to Talk so Your Doctors Will Listen*. New York: Oxford University Press.

Hughes, L., Whittlesea, C. and Luscombe, D. (2002). Patients' knowledge and perceptions of side effects of OTC medication, *Journal of Clinical Pharmacy and Therapeutics*, 27, 243–8.

Hybels, S. and Weaver, R. (1998). *Communicating Effectively*, 5th edn. Boston, MA: McGraw-Hill.

International Medical Benefit/Risk Foundation (IMBRF) (1993). *Improving Patient Information and Education on Medicines*. Geneva: IMBRF.

Jackson, L. (1992). Information complexity and medical communication: the effects of technical language and amount of information in a medical message, *Health Communication*, 4, 197–210.

Jackson, L.D. and Duffy, B.K. (eds) (1998). *Health Communication Research: A Guide to Developments and Directions*. London: Greenwood Press.

Jadad, A.R. (1999). Promoting partnerships: challenges for the Internet age, *British Medical Journal*, 319, 761–4.

Jenkins, V.A., Fallowfield, L.J. and Saul, J. (2001). Information needs of patients with cancer: results from a large study in UK cancer centres, *British Journal of Cancer*, 84, 48–51.

Jenkins, V.A., Fallowfield, L.J. and Poole, K. (2001). Are members of multidisciplinary teams in breast cancer aware of each other's informational roles?, *Quality in Health Care*, 10, 70–5.

Jenz, N.K. and Becker, M.H. (1984). The Health Belief Model: a decade later, *Health Education Quarterly*, 11, 1–47.

Joffe, S., Cook, E.F., Clearly, P.D., Clark, J.W. and Weeks, J.C. (2001). Quality of informed consent in cancer clinical trials: a cross sectional survey, *Lancet*, 358, 1772–7.

Johnson, A. and Sandford, J. (2004). Written and verbal information versus verbal information only for patients being discharged from acute hospital settings to home: a systematic review, *Health Education Research*. 30 November, p. 1.

Johnson, D.W. and Johnson, F.P. (1987). *Joining Together: Group Theory and Group Skills*, 3rd edn. Englewood Cliffs, NJ: Prentice-Hall.

Jones, S.E. and Yarbrough, A.E. (1985). A naturalistic study of the meanings of touch, *Communication Monographs*, 52, 19–56.

Kane, R.L., Ouslander, J.G. and Abbrass, I.B. (1994). *Essentials of Clinical Geriatrics*. New York: McGraw-Hill.

Kar, S.B. Alcalay, R. and Alex, S. (2001). *Health Communication: A Multicultural Perspective*. London: Sage

Katz, J., Peberdy, A. and Douglas, J. (2000). *Promoting Health Knowledge and Practice*, 2nd edn. Milton Keynes: Open University Press.

Katzman, E.M. and Roberts, J.I. (1988). Nurse–physician conflicts as barriers to the enactment of nursing roles, *Western Journal of Nursing Research*, 10, 576–90.

Kenny, T., Wilson, R.G., Purves, I.N., Clark, J., Newton, L.D., Newton, D.P. and Moseley, D.V. (1998). A PIL for every ill? Patient information leaflets (PILs): a review of past, present and future use, *Family Practice*, 15, 471–9.

Kerzman, H., Baron-Epel, O. and Toren, O. (2005). What do discharged patients know about their medication?, *Patient Education & Counselling*, 3, 276–82.

Kim, P., Eng, T.R., Deering, M.J. and Maxfield, A. (1999). Published criteria for evaluating health related web sites: review, *British Medical Journal*, 318, 647–9.

Kimmel, S.R. and Wolfe, R.M. (2005). Communicating the benefits and risks of vaccines, *The Journal of Family Practice*, 54, 51–7.

Kitching, J.B. (1990). Patient information leaflets: the state of the art, *Journal of the Royal Society of Medicine*, 83, 298–300.

Kleinke, C.L. (1986). Gaze and eye contact: a research review, *Psychological Bulletin*, 100, 78–100.

Knapp, M. and Hall, J. (1997). *Nonverbal Communication in Human Interaction*, 4th edn. Fort Worth, TX: Harcourt Brace College Publishers.

Knapp, P.R., Raynor, D.K. and Berry, D.C. (2004). Comparison of two methods of presenting risk information to patients about side effects of medicines, *Quality and Safety in Health Care*, 13, 176–80.

Knobel, R.J. (1983). Health promotion and disease prevention: improving health while conserving resources, *Family and Community Health*, 1, 16–27.

Kreps, G.L. (2003). The impact of communication on cancer risk incidence, morbidity, mortality, and quality of life, *Health Communication*, 15, 161–9.

Kreps, G.L., Bonaguro, E.W. and Query, J.L. (1998). The history and development of the field of health communication research, in L.D. Jackson and B.K. Duffy (eds), *Health Communication Research: A Guide to Developments and Directions*. London: Greenwood Press.

Kreuter, M.W. and Holt, C.L. (2001). How do people process health information? Applications in an age of individualized communication, *Current Directions in Psychological Science*, 10, 206–9.

Kreuter, M.W., Oswald, D.L., Bull, F.C. and Clark, E.M. (2000). Are tailored health education materials always more effective than non-tailored materials?, *Health Education Research*, 15, 305–15.

Kreuter, M.W., Strecher, V.J. and Glassman, B. (1999). One size does not fit all: the case for tailoring print materials, *Annals of Behavioral Medicine: A Publication of the Society of Behavioral Medicine*, 21, 276–83.

Kubler-Ross, E. (1969). *On Death and Dying*. New York: Macmillan.

Langewitz, W.A., Eich, P., Kiss, A. and Wossmer, B. (1998). Improving communication skills: a randomised controlled behaviourally oriented intervention study for residents in internal medicine, *Psychosomatic Medicine*, 60, 268–76.

Larson, D.G. and Tobin, D.R. (2000). End of life conversations: evolving practice and theory, *Journal of American Medical Association*, 284, 1573–8.

Latter, S. and Courtenay, M. (2004) Effectiveness of nurse prescribing: a review of the literature, *Journal of Clinical Nursing*, 13, 26–32.

Leigh, H. and Reiser, M.F. (1986). Comparison of theoretically-oriented and patient-oriented behavioural science courses, *Journal of Medical Education*, 61, 169–74.

Levy, J.A. and Strombeck, R. (2002). Health benefits and risks of the Internet, *Journal of Medical Systems*, 26, 495–510.

Ley, P. (1973). Communication in a clinical setting, *British Journal of Orthodontics*, 1, 173–7.

Ley, P. (1988). *Communicating with Patients*. London: Croom Helm.

Ley, P. and Llewellyn, S. (1995). Improving patients' understanding, recall, satisfaction and compliance, in A. Broome and S. Llewellyn (eds), *Health Psychology: Process and Application*, 2nd edn. London: Chapman and Hall.

Lipkus, I.M., Samsa, G. and Rimer, B.K. (2001). General performance on a numeracy scale among highly educated samples, *Medical Decision Making*, 21, 37–44.

Lister-Sharpe, D., Chapman, S., Stewart-Brown, S. and Sowden, A. (1999). *Health Promoting Schools and Health Promotion in Schools: Two Systematic Reviews*. York: NHS Centre for Reviews and Dissemination.

Livingstone, J., Axton, R.A., Mennie, M., Gilfallan, A. and Brock, D.J. (1993). A preliminary trial of couples screening for cystic fibrosis: designing an appropriate information leaflet, *Clinical Genetics*, 43, 57–62.

Lloyd, M. and Bor, R. (1996). *Communication Skills for Medicine*. Edinburgh: Churchill Livingstone.

Lobb, E.A., Butow, P.N., Barratt, A., Meiser, B., Gaff, C., Young, M.A., Haan, E., Suthers, G., Gattas, M. and Tucker, K. (2004). Communication and information giving in high risk breast cancer consultations: influence on patient outcomes, *British Journal of Cancer*, 90, 321–7.

Loewy, E.H. and Loewy, R.S. (2004). *Textbook of Medical Ethics*, 2nd edn. Dordrecht: Kluwer Academic.

Louis, M.R. and Sutton, R.I. (1991). Switching cognitive gears: from habits of mind to active thinking, *Human Relations*, 44, 55–76.

Luker, K., Austin, L., Hogg, C., Ferguson, B. and Smith, K. (1997) Patients' views of nurse prescribing, *Nursing Times*, 93, 515–18.

Luker, K., Austin, L., Hogg, C., Ferguson, B. and Smith, K. (1998). Nurse–patient relationships: the context of nurse prescribing, *Journal of Advanced Nursing*, 28, 235–42.

MacDonald, E. (2004). *Difficult Conversations in Medicine*. Oxford: Oxford University Press.

MacFarlane, J.T., Holmes, W.F. and MacFarlane, R.M. (1997). Reducing reconsultations for acute lower respiratory tract illness with an information leaflet: a randomised controlled study of patients in primary care, *British Journal of General Practice*, 47, 719–22.

Mackie, D.M. and Worth, L.T. (1989). Processing deficits and the mediation of positive affect in persuasion, *Journal of Personality and Social Psychology*, 57, 27–40.

Maguire, P., Fairburn, S. and Fletcher, C. (1986). Consultation skills of young doctors, *British Medical Journal*, 292, 1573–8.

Maguire, P., Fairburn, S. and Fletcher, C. (1989). Consultation skills of young doctors: benefits of feedback training, in M. Stewart and D. Roter (eds), *Communicating with Patients*. London: Sage.

Maibach, E. and Parrott, R.L. (eds) (1995). *Designing Health Messages: Approaches from Communication Theory and Public Health Practice*. Thousand Oaks, CA: Sage.

Malenka, D.J., Baron, J.A., Johansen, S., Wahrenberger, J.W. and Ross, J.M. (1993). The framing effect of relative and absolute risk, *Journal of General Internal Medicine*, 8, 543–8.

Mannes, S.L., Jacobsen, P.B., Garfinkle, K., Gernstein, F. and Redd, W.H. (1993). Treatment adherence difficulties among children with cancer: the role of parenting style, *Journal of Pediatric Psychology*, 18, 47–62.

Marcus, P.M. (2000). Television as a venue for cancer education: the General Hospital experience, *Journal of Cancer Education*, 14, 4.

Markham, I.S. (1998). Ethical and legal issues, *British Medical Bulletin*, 54, 1011–21.

Marks, D.F., Murray, M., Evans, B. and Willig, C. (2000). *Health Psychology: Theory, Research and Practice*. London: Sage.

Marwick, C. (1997). MedGuide: at last a long sought opportunity for patient education about prescribed drugs, *Journal of the American Medical Association*, 277, 949–50.

Mayberry, J.F. and Mayberry, M.K. (1996). Effective instructions for patients, *Journal of Royal College of Physicians*, 30, 205–8.

Mazur, D.J. and Merz, J.F. (1994). Patients' interpretations of verbal expressions of probability: implications for securing informed consent to medical interventions, *Behavioral Science & Law*, 12, 417–26.

McCormick, J. (1996). Medical hubris and the public health: the ethical dimension, *Journal of Clinical Epidemiology*, 49, 619–21.

McElnay, J.C. and McCallion, R. (1998). Adherence and the elderly, in L.B. Myers and R. Midence (eds), *Adherence to Treatment in Medical Conditions*. London: Harwood.

McNeil, B.J., Pauker, S.G., Sox, H.C. and Tversky, A. (1982). On the elicitation of preferences for alternative therapies, *New England Journal of Medicine*, 306, 1259–62.

Meredith, P. (1993). Patient participation in decision-making and consent to treatment: the case of general surgery, *Social Health & Illness*, 15, 315–36.

Meredith, P., Emberton, M., Wood, C. and Smith, J. (1995). Comparison of patients' needs for information on prostate surgery with printed materials provided by surgeons, *Quality in Health Care*, 4, 18–23.

Morgan, M.G. and Lave, L. (1990). Ethical considerations in risk communication practice and research, *Risk Analysis*, 10, 355–8.

Morris, L.A. (1989). Communicating adverse drug effects to patients, *Journal of Clinical Research and Drug Development*, 3, 53–65.

Morrow, N., Hargie, O., Donnelly, H. and Woodman, C. (1993). Why do you ask? A study of questioning behaviour in community pharmacist: client consultations, *International Journal of Pharmacy Practice*, 2, 90–4.

Mossman, J., Boudioni, M. and Slevin, M.L. (1999). Cancer information: a cost-effective intervention, *European Journal of Cancer*, 35, 1587–91.

Mottram, D.R. and Reed, C. (1997). Comparative evaluation of patient information leaflets by pharmacists, doctors and the general public, *Journal of Clinical Pharmacy Therapy*, 22, 127–34.

Moynihan, R., Bero, L., Ross-Degnan, D., Henry, D., Lee, K., Watkins, J., Mah, C. and Soumerai, S. (2000). Coverage by the news media of the benefits and risks of medications, *New England Journal of Medicine*, 342, 1645–9.

Murray, S.L., Holmes, J.G., and Griffin, D.W. (1996) The self-fufilling nature of positive illusions in romantic relationships, *Journal of Personality & Social Psychology*, 71, 1155–80.

National Services Framework (NSF) (2003). *UK National Services Framework for Children*. London: Department of Health.

Natter, H.M. and Berry, D.C. (2005). Effects of presenting the baseline risk when communicating absolute and relative risk reductions, *Psychology, Health & Medicine*, 10, 326–34.

Newton, L., Newton, D., Clark, J., Kenny, T., Moseley, D., Purves, I. and Wilson, R. (1998). Patient information leaflets: producing understandable PILs, *Journal of Information Science*, 24, 167–81.

Noble, L.M. (1998). Doctor–patient communication and adherence to treatment, in L.B. Myers and K. Midence (eds), *Adherence to Treatment in Medical Conditions*. Amsterdam: Harwood Academic.

Northouse, L.L. and Northouse, P.G. (1998). *Health Communication: Strategies of Health Professionals*. London: Pearson Education.

Nussbaum, J.F., Ragan, S. and Whaley, B. (2003). Children, older adults and women: impact on provider–patient interaction, in T.L. Thompson, A.M. Dorsey, K.I. Miller and R. Parrott (eds), *Handbook of Health Communication*. Mahwah, NJ: Lawrence Erlbaum Associates.

Nutbeam, D. (1998). *Health Promotion Glossary*. Geneva: World Health Organization. Available at www.who.int/hpr/docs/glossary.pdf

O'Connor, A.M. and Edwards, A. (2001). The role of decision aids in promoting evidence-based patient choice, in A. Edwards and G. Elwyn (eds), *Evidence-based Patient Choice: Inevitable or Impossible?* Oxford: Oxford University Press.

O'Connor, A.M., Legare, F. and Stacey, D. (2003). Risk communication in practice: the contribution of decision aids, *British Journal of Psychology*, 327, 736–40.

Oberle, K. and Hughes, D. (2001). Doctors' and nurses' perceptions of ethical problems in end of life decisions, *Journal of Advanced Nursing*, 33, 707–15.

Office of National Statistics (ONS) (2004). *Individuals Accessing the Internet: National Statistics Omnibus Survey*. London: Office for National Statistics. Available at www.statistics.gov.uk/.

Ong, L.M., de Haes, J.C., Hoos, A.M. and Lammes, F.B. (1995). Doctor–patient communication: a review of the literature, *Social Science and Medicine*, 40, 903–18.

Paling, J. (2004). *Helping Patients Understand Risks*. Gainsville, FL: The Risk Communication Institute.

Parker, M. (2004). Judging capacity: paternalism and the risk-related standard, *Journal of Law and Medicine*, 11, 482–91.

Parker, M., Wilkie, A., Ashcroft, R. and Kent, A. (2004). Ethical review of research into rare genetic disorders, *British Medical Journal*, 329, 288–9.

Payne, S., Large, A., Jarrett, N. and Turner, P. (2000). Written information given to patients and families by palliative care nurses: a national survey, *Lancet*, 355, 1792.

Peersman, G., Harden, A. and Oliver, S. (1998). *Effectiveness of Health Promotion Interventions in the Workplace*. London: Health Education Authority.

Petrie, K.J. and Wessely, S. (2002). Modern worries, new technology and medicine, *British Medical Journal*, 324, 690–1.

Pettigrew, L.S. and Logan, R. (1987). The health care context, in C.R. Berger and S.H. Chaffee (eds), *Handbook of Communication Science*. Newbury Park, CA: Sage.

Petty, R. and Cacioppo, J. (1986). *Communication and Persuasion: Central and Peripheral Routes to Attitude Change*. New York: Springer Verlag.

Petty, R.E., Weneger, D.T. and Fabrigar, L.R. (1997). Attitudes and attitude change, *Annual Review of Psychology*, 48, 609–47.

Post, D.M., Cegala, D.J. and Miser, W.F. (2002). The other half of the whole: teaching patients to communicate with physicians, *Family Medicine*, 34, 344–52.

Prigerson, H.G. (1992). Socialisation to dying: the social determinants of death acknowledgement and treatment among terminally ill geriatric patients, *Journal of Health & Social Behaviour*, 33, 378–95.

Ptacek, J.T. and Eberhardt, T.L. (1996). The patient–physician relationship: breaking bad news; a review of the literature, *Journal of American Medical Association*, 276, 6496–502.

Raynor, D.K. (1998). The influence of written information on patient knowledge and adherence to treatment, in L.B. Myers and K. Midence (eds), *Adherence to Treatment in Medical Conditions*. Amsterdam: Harwood Academic.

Raynor, D.K. (2001). PILS: kill or cure? *Pharmacy Business and Practice*, May, 116–18.

Raynor, D.K. and Knapp, P.R. (2000) Do patients see, read and retain new mandatory medicine information leaflets, *Pharmacy Journal*, 264, 268–70.

Redman, S., Spencer, E.A. and Sanson-Fisher, R.W. (1990). The role of the mass media in changing health-related behaviour, *Health Promotion International*, 5, 85–101.

Richardson, D.P. (2005). The scientific substantiation of health claims with particular reference to the grading of evidence and consumer understanding, *Food Science and Technology Bulletin: Functional Foods*, 2, 39–48.

Richardson, D.P., Affertsholt, T., Asp, N.-G., Bruce, A., Grossklaus, R., Howlett, J., Pannemans, D., Ross., R., Verhagen, H. and Viechtbauer, V. (2003). PASSCLAIM: synthesis and review of existing processes, *European Journal of Nutrition*, 42, 96–111.

Roberts, R., Towell, T. and Golding, J.F. (2001). *Foundations in Health Psychology*. Basingstoke: Palgrave.

Rogers, E.M. (1996). The field of health communication today: an up-to-date report, *Journal of Health Communication*, 1, 15–23.

Rogers, E.M. and Kincaid, D.L. (1981). *Communication Networks: Toward a Paradigm for Research*. New York: Free Press.

Rogers, R.W. (1975). A protection motivation theory of fear appeals and attitude change, *Journal of Psychology*, 91, 93–114.

Rosenblum, N., Wetzel, M., Platt, O., Daniels, S., Crawford, J. and Rosenthal, R. (1994). Predicting medical student success in a clinical clerkship by rating students' non-verbal behaviour, *Archives of Pediatric and Adolescent Medicine*, 148, 213–19.

Rosenstock, I.M. (1966). Why people use health services, *Millbank Memorial Foundation Quarterly*, 44, 94–124.

Rosenstock, I.M. (1974). The Health Belief Model and preventative health behaviour, *Health Education Monographs*, 2, 354–6.

Roter, D.L. (2000). The outpatient medical encounter and elderly patients, *Clinical Geriatric Medicine*, 16, 95–107.

Roter, D.L. and Hall, J.A. (1989). Studies of doctor–patient interaction, *Annual Review of Public Health*, 10, 163–80.

Roter, D.L. and Hall, J.A. (1992). *Doctors Talking with Patients/Patients Talking with Doctors*. Westport, CT: Auburn House.

Roter, D.L. and Hall, J.A. (2004). Physician gender and patient-centred communication: a critical review of empirical research, *Annual Review of Public Health*, 25, 497–519.

Roter, D.L., Hall, J.A., Merisca, R., Nordstrom, B., Cretin, D. and Svarstad, B. (1998). Effectiveness of interventions to improve patient compliance: a meta-analysis, *Medical Care*, 36, 1138–61.

Roter, D.L., Stashefsky-Margalit, R. and Rudd, R. (2001). Current perspectives on patient education in the US, *Patient Education & Counselling*, 44, 79–86.

Rutter, D. and Quine, L. (2002). *Changing Health Behaviour: Intervention and Research with Social Cognition Models*. Milton Keynes: Open University Press.

Rutter, M., Maughan, B., Mortimore, P. and Ouston, J. (1979). *Fifteen Thousand Hours*. London: Open Books.

Ryan, P.Y. (1992). Perceptions of the most helpful nursing behaviours in home-care hospice setting: caregivers and nurses, *American Journal of Hospice & Palliative Care*, 9, 22–31.

Schmidt, C. and Brewer, N. (2000). Effects of mood and emotion on juror processing and judgements, *Australian Journal of Psychology*, 52 (2000 supplement), M. Donaghue, M. Innes and I. Waller (eds). Australian Psychological Society, Carlton, Victoria.

Schneider, C.E. (1998). *The Practice of Autonomy: Patients, Doctors & Medical Decisions*. Oxford: Oxford University Press.

Schofield, T. (2004). Introduction, in E. MacDonald (ed.), *Difficult Conversations in Medicine*. Oxford: Oxford University Press.

Schou, K.C. and Hewison, J. (1999). *Experiencing Cancer*. Buckingham: Open University Press.

Schriver, K.A. (1997). *Dynamics in Document Design*. Chichester: John Wiley.

Schultz, E.A. (1998). Informed consent: an overview, *CRNA: The Clinical Forum for Nurse Anaesthetists*, 9, 2–9.

Schwartz, L.M., Woloshin, S., Black, W.C. and Welch, H.G. (1997). The role of numeracy in understanding the benefit of screening mammography, *Annals of Internal Medicine*, 127, 966–72.

Schwarzer, R. (1992). Self-efficacy in the adoption and maintenance of health behaviours: theoretical approaches and a new model, in R. Schwartzer (ed.), *Self-efficacy: Thought Control of Action*. Washington, DC: Hemisphere.

Segrin, C. and Flora, J. (2000). Poor social skills are a vulnerability factor in the development of psychological problems, *Human Communication Research*, 26, 489–514.

Semple, C.J. and McGowan, B. (2002). Need for appropriate written information for patients with particular reference to head and neck cancer, *Journal of Clinical Nursing*, 11, 585–93.

Shannon, C.E. and Weaver, W. (1949). *The Mathematical Theory of Communication*. Champaign, IL: University of Illinois Press.

Sharpe, M., Mayou, R., Seagroatt, V., Surawy, C., Warwick, H., Bulstrode, C., Dawber, R. and Lane, D. (1994). Why do doctors find some patients difficult to help?, *Quarterly Journal of Medicine*, 87, 187–93.

Sheeran, P. and Abraham, C. (1996). The Health Belief Model, in M. Conner and P. Norman (eds), *Predicting Health Behaviours*. Milton Keynes: Open University Press.

Sheridan, S.L. and Pignone, M. (2002). Numeracy and the medical students' ability to interpret data, *Effective Clinical Practice*, 5, 35–40.

Signorelli, N. (1993). *Mass Media Images and Impact on Public Health: A Sourcebook*. Westport, CT: Greenwood Press.

Simpson, M., Buckman, R., Stewart, M., Maguire, P., Lipkin, M., Novack, D. and Till, J. (1991). Doctor–patient communication: the Toronto consensus statement, *British Medical Journal*, 303, 1385–7.

Skelton, J. and Hobbs, F. (1999). Concordancing: use of language based research in medical communication, *Lancet*, 353, 108–11.

Skinner, C.S., Campbell, M.K., Rimer, B.K., Curry, S. and Prochaska, J.O. (1999). How effective is tailored print communication?, *Annals of Behavioral Medicine*, 21, 290–8.

Sleight, P. (1995). Teaching communication skills: part of medical education?, *Journal of Human Hypertension*, 9, 67–9.

Sless, D. (2001). Usable written information for patients, *Medical Journal of Australia*, 174, 557–8.

Sless, D. and Wiseman, R. (1994). *Writing about Medicines for People: Usability Guidelines and Glossary for Consumer Product Information*. Canberra: AGPS.

Smith, E. and Mackie, D. (2000). *Social Psychology*, 2nd edn. Philadelphia, PA: Psychology Press.

Sque, M. and Payne, S. (in press). *Organ Donors and Their Families: Psychological and Social Concerns*. Maidenhead: Open University Press.

Squirer, R.W. (1990). A model of empathic understanding and adherence to treatment regimens in practitioner–patient relationships, *Social Science & Medicine*, 30, 325–39.

Stetz, K., McDonald, J.C. and Compton, K. (1996). Needs and experiences of family caregivers during marrow transplantation, *Oncology Nursing Forum*, 23, 1422–7.

Stewart, R.B. (1990). Polypharmacy in the elderly: a fait accomplice?, *The Annals of Pharmacotherapy*, 24, 321–4.

Stewart, C. and Cash, W. (2000). *Interviewing: Principles and Practice*, 9th edn. Boston, MA: McGraw-Hill.

Stewart, M.A. (1995). Effective physician–patient communication and health outcomes: a review, *Canadian Medical Association Journal*, 152, 1423–33.

Straus, S.E. (2002). Individualizing treatment decisions: the likelihood of being helped or harmed, *Evaluation and the Health Professions*, 25, 210–24.

Street, R.L. (2003) Communication in medical encounters: an ecological perspective, in T.L. Thompson, A.M. Dorsey, K.I. Miller and R. Parrott (eds), *Handbook of Health Communication*. Mahwah, NJ: Lawrence Erlbaum Associates.

Stroebe, W. (2000). *Social Psychology and Health*, 2nd edn. Milton Keynes: Open University Press.

Theodorson, S.A. and Theodorson, G.R. (1969). *A Modern Dictionary of Sociology*. New York: Crowell.

Thompson, T.L. (1998). The patient/health professional relationship, in L.D. Jackson and B.K. Duffy (eds), *Health Communication Research: A Guide to Developments and Directions*. London: Greenwood Press.

Timmermans, D. (1994). The roles of experience and domain of expertise in using numerical and verbal probability terms in medical decisions, *Medical Decision Making*, 14, 146–56.

Tones K. (1998). Health promotion: empowering choice, in L.B. Myers and K. Midence (eds), *Adherence to Treatment in Medical Conditions*. Amsterdam: Harwood Academic.

Tones, K. (1999). The health promoting school: some reflections on evaluation, *Health Education Research*, 11, i–viii.

Tones, K. and Tilford, S. (2001). *Health Promotion: Effectiveness, Efficiency and Equity*, 3rd edn. Cheltenham: Nelson Thornes.

Trask, R.L. (1998). *Language: The Basics*, 2nd edn. London: Routledge.

Traynor, K. (2002). Drug information leaflets for consumers need improvement, FDA says, *American Journal of Health Systems Pharmacy*, 59, 1498–501.

Tufnell, D.J., Nutall, K., Raistrick, J. and Jackson, T.L. (1994). Use of translated written material to communicate with non-English speaking patients, *British Medical Journal*, 309, 992.

Turner, P. and Williams, C. (2002). Informed consent: patients listen and read, but what information do they retain?, *The New Zealand Medical Journal*, 115, 1–7.

Van der Waal, M.A.E., Casparie, A.F. and Lako, C.J. (1996). Quality of care: a comparison of preferences between medical specialists and patients with chronic diseases, *Social Science & Medicine*, 42, 643–9.

Wallace, L. and Lennon, E.S. (2004). American Academy of Family Physicians patient education materials: can patients read them?, *Family Medicine*, 36, 571–4.

Walther, J.B. (1996). Computer mediated communication: impersonal, interpersonal and hyperpersonal interaction, *Communication Research*, 23, 23–43.

Wassmer, E., Minnar, G., Aal, N.A., Atkinson, M., Gupta, E., Yuen, S. and Rylance, G. (2004). How do paediatricians communicate with children and parents?, *Acta Paediatrica*, 93, 1501–6.

West, C. (1983). 'Ask me no questions . . .': An analysis of queries and replies in physician–patient dialogues, in S. Fisher and A.D. Todd (eds), *The Social Organisation of Doctor–Patient Communication*. Washington, DC: Center of Applied Linguistics.

White, P., Smith, H., Webley, F. and Frew, A. (2004). A survey of the quality of information leaflets on hayfever available from general practices and community pharmacies, *Clinical & Experimental Allergy*, 34, 1438–43.

Whitte, P., Kreps, G.L. and Eastin, M.S. (2005). Creating a framework for online cancer services research to facilitate timely and interdisciplinary applications, *Journal of Medical Internet Research*, 7, 34.

Williams, M.V., Parker, R.M., Baker, D.W., Parikh, N.S., Pitkin, K., Coates, W.C. and Nurss, J.R. (1995). Inadequate functional health literacy among patients in two public hospitals, *Journal of American Medical Association*, 274, 1677–82.

Williams, O.A. (1993). Patient knowledge of operative care, *Journal of the Royal Society of Medicine*, 86, 328–31.

Williams, S., Weinman, J. and Dale, J. (1998). Doctor–patient communication and patient satisfaction: a review, *Family Practice*, 15, 480–92.

Wilson, M., Robinson, E.J., Blenkinsopp, A. and Panton, R. (1992). Customers' recall of information given in community pharmacies, *International Journal of Pharmacy Practice*, 1, 52–9.

Windahl, S. and Signitzer, B. (1992). *Using Communication Theory: An Introduction to Planned Communication*. London: Sage.

Witte, K. (1995). Fishing for success: using the persuasive health message framework to generate effective health campaigns, in E. Maibach and R.L. Parrott (eds), *Designing Health Messages: Approaches from Communication Theory and Public Health Practice*. Thousand Oaks, CA: Sage.

Wolff, F., Marsnik, N., Tracey, W. and Nichols, R. (1983). *Perceptive Listening*. New York: Holt, Rinehart and Winston.

World Health Organization (WHO) (1997). *Promoting Health through Schools: Report of a WHO Expert Committee on Comprehensive School Health Education and Promotion*. Geneva: World Health Organization.

Wright, P. (1998). Designing healthcare advice for the public, in F. Durso (ed.), *Handbook of Applied Cognition*. Chichester: John Wiley.

Yalom, I.D. (1995). *The Theory and Practice of Group Psychotherapy*, 4th edn. New York: Basic Books.

Ziebland, S., Chapple, A., Dumelow, C., Evans, J., Prinjha, S. and Rozmovits, L. (2004). How the Internet affects patients' experience of cancer: a qualitative study, *British Medical Journal*, 328, 564.

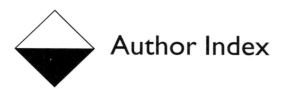

Author Index

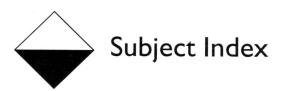

Subject Index